# HOPE HELP & HEALING

## TRAVELING FOR TREATMENT IN CHINA

by

Ruth E. Lycke & Karen Lauritzen

authorHOUSE®

*AuthorHouse*™
*1663 Liberty Drive, Suite 200*
*Bloomington, IN 47403*
*www.authorhouse.com*
*Phone: 1-800-839-8640*

*First published by AuthorHouse   12/31/2007*

*ISBN: 978-1-4343-5402-0 (sc)*

*Library of Congress Control Number: 2007909879*

*Printed in the United States of America*
*Bloomington, Indiana*

*This book is printed on acid-free paper.*

# TABLE OF CONTENTS

# PREFACE

Your body is the only one you have and as such should be handled with care. Many times it takes an "event", the all-encompassing word many to call a life threatening illness, in our lives to help us understand this. I experience the "event" of a stroke and am a stroke survivor. I want to thank you for taking this time to read and learn from the phrase, "It is not what you know that matters, but what you are willing to learn".

I *hope* that this book will bring you the *help* you need in finding and experiencing the *healing* you deserve!

Ruth

---

I have witnessed first -hand the benefits of whole body healing as I visited my son during his TCM (Traditional Chinese Medicine) treatment. As a family member of a loved one and a medical social worker, I watched in wonder as seemingly miraculous healing occurred using age-old Chinese medicine. I invite you to read this book and glean from it nuggets of wisdom, truth, and hope.

This book was published in Garamond 14 point type with additional spacing to make it easier to read. The purpose in choosing this type was to slow down processing a large amount of information. We hope the reader will find this helpful.

Karen

# 简介

# INTRODUCTION

China, 0ften called "Beautiful China" -- a country steeped in culture and history yet not thought of as a nation that delivers some of the finest medical care in the world. China is on the map as a leader in the global economy, host for the 2008 Olympic Games and the nation with the largest population and the oldest civilization in the world. China is a leading economic powerhouse and hub for medical treatment and tourism. With the surge to improve the Chinese infrastructure, state of the art facilities have been built and staffed with world-renowned physicians. Many people know China to be a center for rejuvenation promised by acupuncture, Chinese medicines and Chinese massage. These specialties are just a small part of Traditional Chinese Medicine offered and are only the tip of a unique combination age-old and cutting edge medical options China offers. In addition, TCM (Traditional Chinese Medicine) and top class medical expertise are offered at very competitive prices. New Chinese corporate hospitals attract foreign patients for high-end surgeries such as Cardiac Bypass or a Knee/Hip Replacement. Five thousand year old Traditional Chinese Medicine exists side by side with these state of the art specialties.

# 1

# 中医治疗方法

# CHINESE MEDICAL APPROACH

# What is different about the Chinese approach?

In Chinese medicine, the body is viewed as a whole. The result is treatment that reflects that observation. An individual is seen as a composite of emotional, spiritual and physical. One part of the body cannot be treated without affecting the rest So often in medicine we look for the quick fix and pop a pill that will cure all our ills. Chinese medicine acknowledges that we are a much more complicated being. Our failure to understand this often ends up with results we either didn't fully expect. In other words, many times the operation or treatment is a complete success and yet we don't find the recovery we seek.

Treatment is often referred to the application of medical care to cure disease, heal injuries, or ease symptoms or a particular remedy, procedure, or technique for curing or alleviating a disease, injury, or a condition.

Treatment goes beyond science. In other words, it is not enough to do the right things physically, there must also believe in the steps. Removing someone's gallbladder may seem like a simple surgical procedure. The patient is told they must have this surgery or risk additional pain and suffering or worse. With this information, they make the decision to go ahead and trust in their surgeon to proceed. When the surgeon removes the diseased organ and sews up the patient their job in treating that single part of the person is complete. The patient leaves the hospital with discharge instructions and

3

a prescription and an appointment for a follow-up. A visit to the doctor is made to be certain that healing is continuing.

---

**"I couldn't have wished for a nicer or more professional group of people to look after me. The treatment was absolutely wonderful."**

**June N.**

---

As a medical professional and patient, Ruth has seen and experienced treatment first hand. Whether it's emergency medicine, surgery, or long term care, she has had the opportunity to participate and receive care on both sides of the planet and can say without hesitation there is a huge difference. The difference is not in the technology or skill that is available and practiced, but in the environment in which it is applied.

Ruth learned first hand through her own rehabilitation how valuable good health and medical care is to those in need. The last thing to question is price or quality. Unfortunately, with the sky rocketing costs of surgical and medical care in the United States, more people are searching the globe for solutions. With the technology and training available worldwide, and with ease of travel, we now have vistas that bring new options and, with it, hope. Current statistics show that over 43 million Americans are currently uninsured and between 1997 and 2003 there was a 5.5 percent decrease in the number of hospitals registered in the U.S. Following this trend over 550,000 Americans left the U.S. in order to seek health care elsewhere. The development and growth of a new industry referred to as medical tourism can meet that need.

## What exactly is medical tourism?

Medical tourism can be broadly defined as the provision of cost effective private medical care in collaboration with the tourism industry for patients needing surgical or other forms of specialized treatment. In other words, providing lower cost health care allows a patient to not only travel for healthcare, but have a brief vacation as well. Health care tourism is now beginning to be facilitated by the corporate sector as well as the tourism industry, both private and public. As large companies see health care costs spiral out of sight, they too are looking for ways to offer more value to their employees.

Chinese medical treatment takes medical tourism to a new level. As a result of the numbers of new hospitals built, wait time for any treatment is much lower in China than in anywhere else in the world. In fact, the numbers of hospitals in the U.S. actually decreased last year and there is a recognized nursing shortage that is now increasing. These facts combined with so many other real life situations help to explain why so many people are looking for other health alternatives.

Medical treatment is often not just an elective option, but a medical necessity. Unnecessary delays for a treatment of a condition often cause critical complications. Waiting time can compromise the health of the client while they await a procedure. It is not uncommon to spend weeks, if not months, between doctor visits seeking approval or referrals. We have to become sensitive to what are often urgent medical concerns. Looking for the program that can deliver needed medical services to the patient desperately needing treatment in weeks rather than months is now available in China.

## Am I a candidate for Chinese Medical treatment?

Chinese Medical treatment can be divided into the following categories:

- Traditional Chinese Medicine
- Cardiac Medicine & Surgery
- Orthopedic Medicine& Surgery
- Cosmetic Medicine & Surgery
- Female Medicine & Surgery
- Eye, Ear, Nose and Throat Medicine & Surgery
- Urinary and Male Medicine & Surgery
- General Medicine & Surgery

If you are in need of any of these services and are seeking quality of care and a relaxed environment, then you are a candidate for Chinese medical treatment.

## Do you want to get the best medical treatment at the best value?

China Connection, the only and exclusive medical tourism program in China, has established key alliances with each of the specialties listed to provide the best treatments and prices available. It's not enough to have need. There are other things to consider: high quality medical care, value in price, decreased wait time for treatment, adequate rehabilitation and recovery time, and an administrator and company who knows first hand what patients seek

## Are you seeking medical treatment for any of the listed conditions?

Traditional Chinese Medicine for patients seeking treatment outside the U.S., including but not limited to:

⇒ Alzheimer's Disease

⇒ Anxiety

⇒ Asthma

⇒ Arthritis

⇒ Allergies

⇒ Backache

⇒ Bels Palsy

⇒ Bronchitis

⇒ Coughs

⇒ Chest Pain (muscle)

⇒ Chronic Fatigue

⇒ Constipation

⇒ Dizziness

⇒ Depression

⇒ Digestive Upsets

⇒ Gastric Pain

⇒ Hay Fever

⇒ Hair Loss

⇒ Heavy Periods

⇒ Habitual Miscarriages

⇒ Hypertension

⇒ Insomnia

⇒ Irritable Bowl Syndrome

⇒ Infertility

⇒ Impotence

⇒ Irregular Menstruation

⇒ Low Sperm Count

⇒ Menopausal Disorders

⇒ Migraine

⇒ MS

⇒ Nervous Disorders

⇒ Over Weight

⇒ Palpitations

⇒ Paralysis

⇒ Parkinson's Disease

⇒ Poor Completion

⇒ Psoriasis

⇒ Period Pain

⇒ RSD

⇒ Stress

⇒ Shingles

⇒ Stroke

⇒ Sport Injury

⇒ Stopping Smoking

⇒ Tennis Elbow

⇒ Tinnitus

⇒ Fatigue

⇒ Urinary Infections

⇒ Urinary Retention

⇒ Varicose Veins

⇒ Vertigo

Western Medicine and Surgery for patients seeking treatment outside the U.S., including but not limited to:

## Bones, Joints & Tendons

- ACL Repair
- Ankle Fusion Operation - Arthodesis
- Broken Ankle - Open Reduction and Fixation
- Bunionectomy
- Carpal Tunnel Decompression
- Discectomy - Slipped Disc
- Dupuytrens Contracture - Partial Fasciectomy
- Epidural
- Femoral Shaft Fracture - Internal Fixation
- Ganglion Excision - Foot
- Ganglion Excision - Wrist
- Hip Replacement

- Knee Arthroscopy
- Knee Replacement
- Radius and Ulna Fracture - Internal Fixation
- Shoulder Arthroscopy
- Shoulder Tendon Repair - Rotator Cuff
- Spinal Fusion
- Spinal Stenosis Operation
- Spine - Total Disc Replacement (TDR)
- Tendon Repair - Achilles Tendon
- Tendon Repair - Extensor
- Tendon Repair - Flexor
- Toe Fusion - Arthodesis
- Toe Nail Removal

## Breast

- Breast - Wide Excision and Axillary Sample
- Breast Biopsy
- Mastectomy
- Mastectomy - Male Subcutaneuos

## Cardiology

- Abdominal or Thoracic Aortic Aneurysm Surgery
- Angioplasty (Balloon & Stent)
- ASD (Atrial Septal Defect) Closure
- Coronary Artery Bypass Graft (CABG) Open Heart Surgery

- PDA (Patent Ductus Arteriosus) Ligation
- Radio Frequency Ablation
- TOF (Total Correction: four abnormality correction)
- Valve Replacement Surgery
- VSD (Ventricular Septal Defect) Closure

## Blood Vessel System

- Aortic Aneurysm
- Axillo-Femoral Bypass
- Femoral Embolectomy
- Femoro-Femoral Bypass
- Femoro-Popliteal Bypass
- Varicose Ulcer Treatment
- Varicose Vein Removal
- Varicose Vein Laser Removal (ELVeS)

## Diagnostics

- 24 hour holter (EKG) monitoring
- Carotid Angiography
- CAT Scan
- Diagnostic Cardiac Catheterization (Coronary Angiogram)
- Echocardiography
- Electrocardiogram (EKG)
- Electrophysiology Testing (Arrhythmia)
- Exercise Echocardiography

- Exercise Stress Testing
- MRI
- Myocardial Biopsy
- Ultrasound
- X-Ray

## Ear, Nose and Throat

- Bronchoscopy - Elective
- Bronchoscopy - Emergency
- Grommet Insertion
- Grommet Removal
- Laryngoscopy and Biopsy
- Maxillary Antral - Sinus Washout
- Myringotomy
- Nasal Polyp Removal
- Parotid Gland Removal - Parotidectomy
- Septoplasty
- Stapedectomy
- Sub mucous Resection - SMR
- Tonsillectomy (Adult)
- Turbinates of Nose - Excision
- Tympanoplasty - Myringoplasty (Adult)

## Eye Surgery

- Cataract Surgery
- LASIK Laser Refraction

- Macular Degeneration
- Retinal Surgery / Vitrectomy

## Female Reproductive System and Pregnancy

- Abcess - Pelvic
- Anterior Repair
- Bartholins Gland Marsupialisation
- Cesarean Section
- Colposuspension
- Cone Biopsy of Cervix
- Dilation and Curettage - D and C
- Hysterectomy - Abdominal
- Hysterectomy - Vaginal
- Laparoscopy
- Laparoscopy and Dye
- Microwave Edometrial Ablation
- Posterior Repair - Prolapse Operation
- Salpingo-oophorectomy - Ectopic Pregnancy
- Sterilization
- Vaginal and Vulval Warts - Removal
- Vulval Lesion Excision

## General Surgery

- Abdomino - Perineal Resection of Rectum
- Abscess - Intra Abdominal
- Abscess - Pelvic

- Abscess - Subphrenic
- Amputation - Above Knee
- Amputation - Below Knee
- Amputation - Toe
- Cholecystectomy - Gall Bladder Removal
- Epididymal Cyst Removal
- Hernia Repair - Epigastric
- Hernia Repair - Femoral
- Hernia Repair - Inguinal
- Hydrocele Operation - Adult
- Pilonidal Sinus
- Spleen Removal - Splenectomy
- Thyroidectomy

## Kidney and Urinary System

- Bladder Outlet Incision
- Cysto-Diathermy
- Cystoscopy
- Nephrectomy - Kidney removal
- Nephrolithotomy - Removal of Kidney stone
- Retrograde Pyelogram
- Ureterolithotomy - Dormia Basket
- Urethroscopy

## Male Reproductive System and Urinary Tract

- Circumcision
- Hydrocele Operation - Adult

- Penis Frenuloplasty
- Prostatectomy
- Vasectomy
- Vasectomy Reversal

## Physical Exams

- Basic Physical Exam
- Comprehensive Physical Exam
- Executive Physical Exam

## Stomach and Bowel

- Abdominal - Perineal Resection of Rectum
- Abscess - Perianal
- Anal Fissure
- Anal Fistula
- Anterior Resection of Rectum
- Appendicectomy
- Colectomy - Total - and Ileostomy
- Colon Polyp Removal
- Colonoscopy
- Colostomy - Defunctioning Loop
- Colostomy Closure - Colorectal Anastomosis
- Gastroscopy
- Hemorrhoid Injection
- Hemorrhoid
- Hemi-Colectomy - Left

- Hemi-Colectomy – Right
- Sigmoid-Colectomy

## COSMETIC

- Breast Augmentation
- Breast Lift
- Breast Reduction
- Buttocks Augmentation (Gluteal Implants)
- Buttocks Lift
- Chemical Peel
- Chin Surgery
- Dermabrasion
- Ear Surgery
- Eyelids
- Face Lift
- Facial Implants
- Facial Line Filling
- Forehead / Brow Lift
- Injectable Fillers
- Liposuction
- Neck Lift
- Nose Surgery
- Spider Veins
- Thigh Lift
- Tummy Tuck
- Upper Arm Lift

# 2

# 中国和

## CHINA &
## CHINA CONNECTION

## Why China Connection?

China Connection works as your medical concierge and facilitates high quality, affordable medical treatment, rehabilitation, and health care tourism in China. We are well versed in what is often referred to as integrated medicine, combining the best of Traditional Chinese Medicine and Western Medicine. We have a full time staff that is American and Chinese, including doctors, nurses and former patients, who are available both in the States as well as China. In addition to medical expertise, we also work to assist clients in arranging and experiencing the rich natural and cultural vistas China offers. Unlike other companies that work only to offer medical tourism in multiple countries to the lowest bidder, China Connection remains focused on a single country. After all, who first integrated medicine? Who took the best Chinese traditional medicine and combined it with technology and the science of western medicine? China. China Connection strives to offer the best medical options available and takes pride in seeing things from a total body perspective. China Connection is unlike any other company. Nothing beats direct experience as President and CEO, Ruth Lycke, can testify. She developed her company after being the first American stroke survivor to seek and receive successful treatment in China. As a result of her experience, she offers a unique point of view to each patient considering medical tourism in China. Ruth spent five months as a rehabilitation patient in China receiving Traditional Chinese Medicine. She experienced nearly a full recovery. She now spends the majority of her time working in her China office, helping clients, including stroke survivors, to recover.    She also coordinates the finest and most cost effective surgery and treatment available. Ruth's recovery has spurred a passion deep within, making it her goal to reach out and help others enjoy the same quality of life she now enjoys. When asked "Why China?" The answer is apparent and can be summed up in another question: "There are students, teachers and masters… to who would you rather entrust your life?"

As a result of her extensive time in China, Ruth has developed direct working relationships with Chinese hospitals and Province governments. She is a former nurse, paramedic, surgical specialist, and clinic manager. Her knowledge and expertise is invaluable. She knows the staff, the doctors in China, the culture and has become a hand's on administrator. This kind of professional relationship, plus an experiential knowledge of the health care system in the U.S and China, assures that the best quality health care services in China are both coordinated and delivered.

---

**"I have no regrets about coming to China."**

**Stephanie T.**

---

Begun in 2005, China Connection has a proven track record of patient satisfaction.  It has delivered and ensured carefully supervised treatment and travel of hundreds of people from the United States, Australia, England, Korea, Singapore, and Japan.

China Connection was established after Ruth suffered a brain stem bleed and stroke and found answers to her rehab questions through Traditional Chinese Medicine in China. She sees treatment and care from the perspective of the patient. Each time she enters a hospital, or clinic she observes the facility, not only from view of a medical professional, but through the eyes of the patient. The kind of knowledge Ruth offers to clients comes, then, from both professional training and real time spent as a patient in China.

## What exactly does China Connection do?

China Connection actively seeks patients worldwide who are candidates for medical tourism. These candidates are carefully screened to ensure a good match for international travel and for the services that are offered. The potential client is not only screened medically, but educated in the protocols of medical procedures abroad.

China Connection offers a full time staff and offices both in the US and China to facilitate timely communication. The China staff works full time in China and has college educated native Chinese, all of whom speak fluent English and are familiar with each medical facility China Connection uses. The U.S. staff works to provide all the documentation necessary to make each trip a successful one. They will assist with medical records transfers, passport, visas, travel information and are a conduit for the client before clients leave the country to travel.

An Informational DVD is sent at the client's request. On line video is also provided for those who have the ability to use it.

U.S. Client Manager Assistance – Unlimited consultation is provided with a qualified personal manager to help each client acquire all the knowledge necessary to experience a successful medical retreat.

Chinese Client Manager Assistant –A Chinese Personal Assistant will be assigned to each client. This individual will be available via phone and be a friend away from home. They will coordinate all client transportation and personal needs. Their services and knowledge are invaluable. Having this contact helps to avoid miscommunication between our respective cultures and better ensures client safety.

Unlimited China Connection Website Access – chinaconnection.cc - Explore the wealth of information on our website. We will also help to guide clients and families through all the specific areas of interest.

Comprehensive Estimate – Receive a thorough estimate Including pricing, hospital information, doctor's resume, doctor's recommendations and hotel accommodations, if applicable.

Detailed Itinerary – A time line of all medical treatment and travel.

Air Travel Arrangements – We offer the assistance of a travel agency that provides competitive airline pricing. We take in consideration of the fastest and most direct routes available. We also know what services are available at overseas facilities and how to use them.

Travel Insurance Opportunities - This package alleviates travel concerns by insuring the client's trip against potential setbacks.

In China Travel Arrangements – We help in coordinating arrival and transportation to and from the airport to hospital and or hotel. Once a client arrives, our drivers handle all bags and transportation from the airport to the medical destination and /or hotel.

Hotel Accommodation Reservations – We provide four and five star hotel access. China Connections has experienced these hotels first hand and can attest to their claims of quality and cleanliness. We highly caution against Internet advertised hotels other than those recommend. Our staff has visited many of the competing hotels surrounding those we recommend. They look great in photos, but often leave much to be desired in person. They speak fluent English and provide western style toilets.

Procedure Treatment Information - To help research your surgical choice, you can review procedure options via helpful on-line links. Although many clients are well informed of their condition, there is always something more to learn. China Connection has on- line links help clients to do research.

Hospital/Doctor Bios - Specific information about the hospitals and doctors is an important aspect to choosing the right facility to perform a procedure. This information will allow a client to make an informed decision about where surgery will be performed and by whom.

Doctor Consultation - On site consultation before surgery. All clients are given VIP preferred treatment throughout their stay. Before discharge from the hospital the doctor also answer specific questions about each client's condition.

Medical Questionnaire Facilitation to Hospital – A complete medical questionnaire form will be forwarded to clients for specific information about medical history. This form will be forwarded to the surgeon or doctor and will help to determine qualifications for the procedure or treatment sought.

Procedure Scheduling - Detailed schedule of surgical events and follow-up services. Unlike many services, a client will not be asked to leave the facility to sit for weeks in a hotel with a nurse for follow up and recuperation. Doctors will not release a client from their care until they are ready to travel. Clients will also have access to many of our recuperation services depending upon specific needs and/or rehab schedule.

Pre-Surgery Consultation in Destination - Before a client commits to surgery, they will have the opportunity to meet with their doctor to confirm their decision to move forward. This meeting will also serve as a discovery process for the doctor to make additional recommendations.

Post Treatment Recuperation Plans - We will discuss plans to either, relax and recuperate, or, to enjoy the interesting attractions a destination offers. This will be contingent upon the type of medical options and the client's individual recovery progress.

Traveler Vaccination Information - Although clients are not required to have vaccinations before traveling to China, we recommend visiting the CDC's website for information about the risks of traveling without proper vaccinations. We strongly suggest their consideration of proper vaccinations.

Passport/Visa Assistance - We will help clients obtain the necessary travel documents for access into and for travel within China.

Transcript Digital Duplication Service - To most effectively receive a firm price quotation abroad, we will help send client transcripts to the hospital. In lieu of submitting their originals, we have affiliates who will digitally copy information to be forwarded overseas without compromising the originals (fee based on quantity).

Financing Opportunities - If clients cannot afford a medical procedure at this time, our affiliates will help to locate a finance company to provide the required money necessary for the medical treatment. In many cases, clients can receive a year's interest free terms if their credit is good.

U.S. Bank Holding Account – If a client did not book their procedure through China Connection, he would be required to send the total amount of procedure costs, in advance, to the hospital. Dealing in cash upfront is standard in China, but several of our facilities work with insurance companies. To help alleviate concerns of fraud, we will allow clients to deposit fees into our U.S. bank account for transfer to their overseas medical facility. Only 10% of funds are initially released and the balance is held until after clients have had the doctor's consultation and have decided to move forward. In the unlikely event that a client decides not to receive treatment, the money will be immediately refunded by China Connection, an American company. This alleviates concerns about collecting from an unknown, overseas bank.

Travel Tips - A helpful PDF resource booklet of information about planning your trip.

Suggesting Reading Material - We'll provide clients with recommendations of books to read and CDs to listen to during their retreat. This information will prove to be beneficial to their psychological well being during recovery.

International Calling Card Outlet - Easy access to calling cards are provided at reduced phone rates to keep in touch with family and friends while away from home (Fee service).

Cell Phone Arrangements - Chinese cell phones and SIM cards to help keep clients in communication with family, friends and overseas contacts (Fee service).

A/C Power Converter Resources - Many of our destinations do not provide access to 110-volt electricity. We provide the information to purchase a power converter and /or adapter to use US appliances.

Currency Converter & Measurement Conversion Calculator - It's important for clients to understand the conversion rates of currency in China. This tool will prove to be essential. China also utilizes the metric system for weights and measures. This calculator will help clients compare our measurement system with those of China.

World Time Information - Use this link to receive information about the time difference between your region in the U.S. or in the world and China.

# 3

在中国独家代理的医院

# EXCLUSIVE HOSPITALS IN CHINA

## I am a candidate for Chinese medical treatment?

The type of surgery or medical experience the client selects will determine the choice of hospital. Each hospital in our system is unique and offers a different service. We offer you an inside look into each of the facilities and they are listed below.

## First Teaching Hospital University of TCM

.................................Traditional Chinese Medicine

## Aimin Weight Loss Hospital

...................................................Weight Loss

## TEDA International Cardiovascular Hospital

.....................Cardiovascular Medicine and Surgery

## TEDA Hospital

............................Orthopedic Medicine and Surgery
.....................Ear, Nose, Throat Medicine and Surgery
..............................Eye Medicine and Surgery
...............................Urinary Medicine and Surgery
....................Male Reproduction Medicine and Surgery
..................Female Reproduction Medicine and Surgery
...............................General Medicine and Surgery
..............................Cosmetic Medicine and Surgery

# TEDA International Cardiovascular Hospital

It is estimated that 13,000 people die of cardiovascular disease, cancer and other chronic diseases every day in China. Nearly 2,400 Americans die of CVD (cardiovascular disease) each day. For Americans that is an average of 1 death every 36 seconds. CVD claims more lives each year than cancer, chronic lower respiratory diseases, accidents and diabetes mellitus combined. Cardiovascular disease has become one of the top killers threatening human lives worldwide. In China, patients needing cardiovascular operations exceed 8,000,000, while currently only less than 80,000 could be done annually.

Cardiovascular procedures require high technology, state-of-the-art equipment, and effective team work in an efficiently managed facility. These requirements make it impossible for ordinary general hospitals to conduct cardiovascular operations and cardiovascular intervention treatment successfully on a large scale. Therefore comprehensive, specialized cardiovascular hospitals are needed to meet these demands. It was determined in China that these hospitals should be accessible nationally in order to operate economically and efficiently.

TEDA is the abbreviation for Tianjin Economic Development Area, which was founded as one of the first 14 state-level development zones approved by State Council in 1984. TEDA, 40 km Eastern to Tianjin City proper, is on the Coast of Bohai Sea, is the close neighbor of Xingang, one of the 10 biggest harbors in the world. It is an economical leader in the Tianjin-Binhai New Area, which is comprised of TEDA, Free-Trade Zone, Tanggu District, Hangu District, Dagang District. More than twenty years after its formation, TEDA has attracted over 4,000 foreign invested enterprises, including such leading multinational companies as MOTOROLA, TOYOTA, YAMAHA, NESTLE, NOVO NORDISK and SAMSUNG, with a total investment of $20 billion U.S dollars. This foreign investment has made it one of the fastest growing areas in China with an annual GDP growth of 30%. It is estimated that the GDP in TEDA will increase at least sixteen times from year 2000 to 2020. An attractive investment environment, a fast-growing economy with convenient transportation as well as an open and pragmatic government make TEDA a bridgehead for Tianjin to accomplish eastward strategic movement and establish an international metropolis-port as well as a legendary pearl at the Bohai Sea economic rim. The central government of China has stated that TEDA, a Tianjin-Bohai New Area, will be developed into the third pole of national economy growth of China, after Shijiazhuang Delta and Yangtze River Delta. This strategic decision provides a greater chance for TEDA's development.

In order to diversify its current economic/social structure, and to solve the supply-demand conflict for cardiovascular operations, TEDA Administrative Commission decided to build  TEDA International Cardiovascular Hospital (TICH). This hospital would open to both the domestic and the international markets in an effort to boost the regional economy and would be the largest cardiovascular hospital in Asia. Dr. LIU Xiaoping, The former Vice-President of Chinese Academy of Medical Sciences and a well-known professor of cardiovascular surgery decided to found a cardiovascular hospital. This hospital would be a new model of management to pave the way for Chinese medical system reformation. This new modern cardiovascular hospital emerged in 2003.

TICH is a publicly owned nonprofit hospital. The construction area of the main building is 76,000 square meters. The initial investment for it totals over $97 million U.S. dollars (¥720 million). It functions as a clinical, teaching and research center with 600 beds, 16 operation rooms, 80 ICU beds, 5 cardiac catheter rooms and 40 CCU beds.

It is equipped with state-of-the-art equipment for diagnosis, treatment and medical research. The equipment includes the latest magnetic resonance imaging (twin speed MRI), multi-slice CT (light speed 16), the new electron beam CT (E-Speed, that is the third installation in the world), ECT, flat plenum equipment for angiography, real-time three dimensional electrocardiography , (just on clinical trial in Mayo Clinic, Johns Hopkins Hospital and Cedars-Sinai Medical Center in USA), high power electronic microscope and a variety of additional advanced medical and research equipment. It is first in the use of automatic tablet counting and dispensing robot in China to improve efficiency, accuracy, and quality of patient medication. The clinical laboratory is also equipped with PAM for high accuracy diagnostic testing. The advanced image storing and transferring system (PACS) and hospital information system (HIS) make it the first domestic paperless and film free hospital and is comparable to other leading hospitals in the world. With the support of HIS, all the outpatient departments use a one-card system where transactions are synchronized. All the advanced management concepts and systems meet the international standards, making TICH not only a leading cardiovascular treatment center and a health service center, but also a training base for cardiovascular clinicians and postgraduate students and a research base for new medicines and new therapies.

TICH comprehensively covers care, teaching, research, and rehabilitation. As a cardiovascular professional hospital, TICH focuses on open-heart surgery and interventional therapy to treat and cure all types of congenital and acquired cardiovascular diseases. The planned capacity of TICH is to conduct over 10,000 cases of surgical operations and 15,000 cases of interventional cardiovascular procedures respectively each year. That surpasses the world records held by Cleveland Clinic in U.S.A., where 7,614 cases of cardiac operation and 12,936 cases of interventional cardiovascular procedure were completed in 2004. TICH is organized into separate treatment sections for all kinds of congenital and acquired cardiovascular diseases, such as congenital heart disease sections, including wards for newborn babies, infants, pre-school children, children of the age group between 7 and 14 as well as adults, and the sections for valve disease, coronary heart disease, great vessel disease, and arrhythmias.

According to market economy principle of classifying consumer groups, all hospital wards are divided into a variety of selections This hospital has small and larger two-bed rooms, small and larger one-bed rooms, suites, and a luxury VIP suite which covers 1,200 square meters including a private elevator. The design of the hospital reflects the patient-oriented concept. Even the smaller, two-bed rooms are equipped not only with air-conditioners, handicap-friendly bathrooms, and Japanese style sliding doors, but also with telephone, flat-screen TV and comfortable bed for each patient. The hospital provides pure water, three meals and one extra meal of fruits without additional cost. In order for ordinary low-income patients to be able to afford hospitalization, they are only charged only $6.75 (¥50) each night in such rooms.

TICH is able to perform all types of cardiovascular surgical procedures, including complex congenital heart disease correction, valve replacement, CABG, great vessel procedures and heart and heart-lung transplantation. All types of interventional cardiovascular procedures, such as PCI, radio frequency catheter ablation, pacemaker embedding and vascular stents for great artery and peripheral arteries are also conducted in TICH. To fully achieve the objectives of care, teaching and research, well equipped medical labs, including a 3,000 square meters central lab with two animal operating rooms, have been set up.

TICH pays maximum attention to optimization of management flow and to domestic and international academic exchange, to master and apply the most advanced technology and to serve the patients better with qualified medical care. One of the greatest benefits to working directly with the TEDA government is being given exclusive access, not only to the TEDA International Cardiovascular Hospital, but to the brand new TEDA Hospital as well.

## TEDA Hospital

The TEDA Hospital, which was established in 1990, began to construct a new and enlarged hospital site by permit of Tianjin Municipal Government in 2005 to meet the demands of the opening of Tianjin Binhai New Area and growing local medical and health care. The new site is situated immediately east of the TEDA International Cardiovascular Hospital, west of Beihai Lu, covering an area of 44,363.24 square meters, with a building area of 78000 square meters, including Comprehensive Medical Treatment Area of 70,000 square meters. Emergency Center of 5,000 square meters, Vocational Diseases Prevention Center of 3,000 square meters. The main in-patient structure is a 12-story building with a total investment value of $72 million U.S dollars (¥530 million Yuan). It was built in accordance with the State standards of Hospitals for Grade I, Category III. It combines the functions of treatment, teaching, research, prevention & health care, and rehabilitation. It currently has 500 beds for patients, 15,000 annual admissions, 2,500 daily out-patient consultations, 8,000 annual operations, and over 150 daily emergency cases. The value of its total medical instruments and equipment comes to more than an additional $19 million U.S. dollars (¥140 million Yuan). The hospital is equipped with a whole-body CT scanner, a MRI scanner, an ECT, various fiber endoscopes, Color Doppler Ultrasonography and other advanced medical devices as well as advanced wholly purified operation rooms, and an Intensive Care Center. Also set up here is a long-distance diagnosis center, forming an emergency system which includes ICU treatment both outside and inside the hospital, capable of admitting injured and ill patients 24 hours a day.

Constantly striving to offer quality services the administration bases the growth of their hospital on scientific research and attracting the leading medical talent. Their focus is on emergency medicine, osteopathic medicine, sports medicine, neurosurgical science, gynecology and obstetrics, otorhinolaryngology, urology, general surgery, digestive medicine, endocrinology and metabolism as major fields to develop. They developed a high capability for prevention, diagnosis and treatment of chemical vocational injuries and diseases.

The TEDA Hospital boasts a team of the best medical experts, many of which have been educated worldwide. It consistently confronts and develops new medical techniques and has formed its own advantages and specialties which are the highest in China: integrated use of blood purification, nutrient and metabolic support, life-support machines, sub hypothermia treatment of acute brain contusions, treatment of hydrocephaly and stroke, operations & treatment of skull defects, athletic injuries, joint replacement, spinal surgery, vessel surgery, minimally invasive operation for larynx, diagnosis and cure of facial nerve paralysis, minimally invasive operations for women, treatment of neonatal diseases, and children's asthma.

TEDA Hospital highlights a patient-centered philosophy of service, facilitating in every treatment aspect safeguards patient interests with the goal of complete recovery.

## First Teaching Hospital of Tianjin University of Traditional Chinese Medicine

A Modern Hospital with a Rich Heritage of Traditional Chinese Medicine

First Teaching Hospital of Tianjin University of Traditional Chinese Medicine was established as Tianjin Municipal Hospital of Traditional Chinese Medicine in 1954. The hospital is the earliest and largest medical facility of Traditional Chinese Medicine, or TCM, in Tianjin. It was named as the National Demonstration TCM Hospital at the Provincial Level, and as one of the one-hundred best Hospitals in China. As a Class A Tianjin Hospital, it is rated as one of a ten best Hospitals in Tianjin and one of three Tianjin Medical Centers. The National Clinical Research Center of

Acupuncture and Moxibustion, the National Special Medical Center of Acupuncture and Moxibustion and the Tianjin Research Institute of Acupuncture and Moxibustion are all situated within this hospital.

The State Education Ministry has defined the subject of Acupuncture and Moxibustion as a keystone science of TCM. The Acupuncture Department, Pediatrics Department and Nephrosis Clinic of the Internal Medicine Department were confirmed as exceptional Departments of National Traditional Chinese Medicine by the State Administration Bureau of Traditional Chinese Medicine. The hospital was designated as the hospital for training and developing medical doctors of Traditional Chinese Medicine and as the National Clinical Testing Center for medications. The hospital is a prestigious, modern hospital, which offers a comprehensive curriculum of Traditional Chinese Medicine and Western Medicine. The hospital and its professional staff are recognized throughout China and the rest of the world for exceptional medical treatment, scientific research and the teaching of Traditional Chinese Medicine.

Many famous professors and doctors work in this hospital including: an academician of the Chinese Academy of Engineering; other experts with outstanding contributions to TCM recognized by the Health Ministry and other experts recognized by the Tianjin Municipal Government as supervisors of medical doctors of Traditional Chinese Medicine. The hospital staff is made up of more than 1,700 to include over 300 professors, associate professors, chief doctors and associate chief doctors. There are over 1300 patient beds in this hospital. The highest number of administrative inpatients at anyone time was approximately 1900 patients. The occupancy rate has been kept over 100% for fourteen years. Amazingly, more than one million outpatients have utilized the services of the hospital each year for nineteen consecutive years. There are more than 30 departments and technical offices and 69 medical clinics in the hospital. The hospital employs more than 1,000 high tech medical instruments for the most advanced level of clinical examination, diagnosis and treatment of disease, illness and other medical conditions. The instruments include: Nuclear Magnetic Resonance Imaging, Whole-body Computed Tomography Imaging, Artificial Kidney Dialysis, Intervertebral Discs Microscopy, Color Ultrasonograph, Skull Color Ultrasonic Doppler System, Automatic Respiratory Machine, Automatic Biochemical Analyzer, Automatic Blood Analyzer, Microelement Examining Machine, Blood Gas Analyzer, Bacteria Analyzer, Electric Gastroscope and Center Monitoring System.

Professor Han Jingxian, the president of this hospital is a scholarly leader and supervisor of medical doctors of Traditional Chinese Medicine. Tianjin municipal government has recognized him as an experimental acupuncture expert and one of the best doctors in Tianjin. The State Council has awarded him a special subsidy for his superior contributions and performance. In addition to his Hospital duties he is the chief director of the Neurology Committee of the Chinese

Committee for Combining Traditional Chinese Medicine and Western Medicine. He also serves as Superintendent of the Tianjin Acupuncture Research Institute. His experimental research of Acupuncture has reached genetic and molecular level. In the midst of all these duties, he maintains a regular schedule of treating hospitalized patients.

Professor Yu Tiecheng, the hospital Party-Committee Secretary, is an effective leader who also serves as a supervisor of medical doctors of Traditional Chinese Medicine. He is the director of the Medical History Documents Research Center, the Research Office of Chinese Medical History, the National Information Digitization Committee of TCM and Chinese Herbs and vice-director of the TCM Culture Branch of the Chinese TCM Committee. His books include "Whole-Subjects of Traditional Chinese Medicine", "Developing a Philosophy for Traditional Chinese Medicine" and "Research on the TCM method of Differentiation of Symptoms and Signs". During his years at the hospital he has been engaged in the research of: medical history documents, TCM culture and the philosophy of TCM.

One of the missions of the hospital is to disseminate the values and advantages of Traditional Chinese Medicine and to cultivate ways of merging TCM and Western Medicine. By combining the advantages of TCM and Western medicine in specialized departments and clinics, the hospital has achieved a remarkable cure rates for many kinds of common clinical diseases, medical conditions and severe emergency cases.

The Acupuncture Department is one of the principle departments for specialized treatments. The National Clinical Research Center of Acupuncture and Moxibustion and the National Special Medical Center of Acupuncture and Moxibustion are both located in the Acupuncture Department. The State Administration Bureau of Traditional Chinese Medicine has confirmed that Acupuncture is the most important keystone subject of TCM at the National and Tianjin levels.

Xing Nao Kai Qiao Therapy or XN KQ is a TCM therapy. This therapy activates the brain and opens the orifices was developed by Prof. Shi Xuemin, an academician of the Chinese Academy of Engineering, XNKQ is well known at home and abroad for its remarkable curative effect in the treatment of strokes. The department is currently conducting research and developing clinical treatments for senile dementia. The Stroke Unit Therapy developed by the Department, is utilized in the treatment of nervous system diseases, cerebral vascular diseases, heart and vascular diseases, asthma, aorto-arteritis and all kinds of pain syndromes. The hospital academic reputation has reached an advanced status at the international level.

The Internal Medicine Department is another of the hospital's-principle areas for specialized treatments. The specialized clinics of the Internal Medicine Department provide treatment of various cardiovascular diseases, kidney diseases, lung diseases, rheumatism, digestive tract diseases, hematopathy, benign and malignant tumors and liver and gall bladder diseases. The clinics are recognized in Tianjin for their remarkable curative treatments.

The Nephrosis Clinic of the Internal Medicine Department was honored by the State Administration Bureau of Traditional Chinese Medicine with the national keystone special science of Traditional Chinese Medicine award. The Clinic has had outstanding success in treating nephritic syndrome, acute nephritis, chronic nephritis, renal insufficiency and uremia.

The Cardiac Disease Clinic of the Internal Medicine Department is tremendously effective in treating coronary heart disease, rheumatic heart disease, arrhythmia and senile diseases, with Traditional Chinese Medicine. It has also developed successful intervention treatment for heart diseases.

The Hematopathy Clinic of the Internal Medicine Department is skilled in the treatment of leukemia, anemia and thrombopenia and other blood diseases.

The Pulmonary Disease Clinic of the Internal Medicine Department is well known for its specialized treatment of pulmonary diseases such as bronchitis and pulmonary emphysema.

The Liver and Gallbladder Disease Clinic of the Internal Medicine Department are skilled in the treatment of familial hepatitis B, chronic hepatitis B and gallbladder diseases.

The Clinic of Rheumatics of the Internal Medicine Department has a very good record of treating some immune system diseases such as rheumatic arthritis, ankylosing spondylitis, systemic lupus erythematosus, sicca syndrome, Behcet's disease and primary vasculitis by combining Chinese Medicine and Western Medicine.

The Digestive Diseases Clinic of the Internal Medicine Department has had remarkable success in treating chronic atrophic gastritis, esophagus, chronic colonitis and irritable bowel syndrome with Traditional Chinese Medicine.

The Clinic of Carcinoma of the Internal Medicine Department treats all kinds of malignant tumors such as lung cancer and stomach cancer with TCM and tridimensional therapy to enhance its curative effects when combined with detoxification and chemotherapy. The Clinic employs a specialized, systemic therapy for treating fever, pain, hydrothorax, and ascites of cancer with traditional Chinese medicine.

The Clinic of Endocrine Disease of the Internal Medicine Department has achieved extraordinary results in treating endocrine diseases such as diabetes and thyroid disease with traditional Chinese medicine.

The Psychosomatic Center has a very positive record in treating prostatitis, psychoneurosis, depression and other mental illnesses.

The Pediatrics Department has also been confirmed as the national keystone special science by State Administration Bureau of Traditional Chinese Medicine and the keystone-developing subject by the Health Bureau of Tianjin Municipal Government. The department is skilled at the treatment of infantile viral myocarditis, nephrosis, epilepsy, cough and asthma, high fever and infantile hyperkinetic syndrome. Its remarkable success has reached advanced levels.

The Surgery Department of Traditional Chinese Medicine is skilled in the treatment of diabetic gangrene, skin and external diseases, piles, mastosis and peripheral vascular diseases.

The Surgery Department of Western Medicine provides the options of general and specialized surgery, such as chest surgery and urinary surgery, as its main focus of treatment. The department also offers surgery for all kinds of medical conditions and diseases as well as micro wound surgery. The doctors utilize specialized instruments such as the abdominoscope, biliary tract scope, cystoscope, urethroscope and prostatic scope in analyzing and providing surgical procedures.

The Extracerebral Department provides surgery and treatment of cerebral hemorrhage and cerebral tumor by applying high tech computer analysis of the brain and highly specialized surgical techniques.

The Intervention Center provides intervention treatment for peripheral vascular and heart diseases such as coronary arteriography, cardiovascular stand implant and cardiac pacemaker implant by utilizing modern instrument.

The Gynecology and Obstetrics Department is very successful in treating hysteromyoma, threatened abortion, endometriosis, pelvic inflammation and other related medical conditions.

The Ophthalmology Department is unique in character and utilizes Traditional Chinese Medicine to treat various eye diseases, retina obstruction, keratopathy glaucoma and cataracts with acupuncture therapy.

The Orthopedics Department applies traditional manipulative treatments for the prolapse of the lumbar intervertebral disc, hyperplasia and all kinds of closed fractures. The department also performs trauma, arthroscopic and lumbar intervertebral discscopic surgery.

The Tuina Department has positive results in treating cervical disease, poliomyelitis crossfoot and progressive myodystrophy with the use Tuina manipulation.

The Dermatology Department is skilled in the treatment of psoriasis, chloasma, acne and venereal disease.

The Otolaryngology Department is proficient in the treatment of chronic nasosinusitis and tympanitis, and other diseases of the nose and throat.

The Stomatology Department has the ability to successfully treat tunica mucosa, oris disease and tooth restoration and cosmetics.

The Rehabilitation Department provides treatment of many chronic diseases including the consequences of stroke, paralysis due to cerebral disease, paraplegia and soft tissues injury by applying the therapy of Tuina, Qigong, exercise and baths with Chinese herbs.

The Emergency Department has an enviable record in saving the lives of persons with multiple organ failure such as heart, respiratory and renal failure. It also is known for its high quality trauma and emergency care. Emergency medicine has reached such an advanced level of efficiency in China that many lives are saved. The Emergency Department of this hospital is the model organization for the International Emergent Salvage Network Hospitals of the Chinese Health Bureau and the Asian Emergency Salvage Center. They provide treatment for severely ill or inured patients with 24 hours service, prompt treatment and modern techniques and instruments.

First Teaching Hospital of Tianjin University of Traditional Chinese Medicine continues to innovate and disseminate knowledge of Traditional Chinese Medicine. In order to introduce Traditional Chinese Medicine to the world, several approaches have been developed for making others aware of their success. The hospital has undertaken the responsibility for training both Chinese and foreign students. More than 3000 doctors and students from 69 countries have received TCM training. The hospital has held 8 International Conferences concerning Clinical Research in Acupuncture, Moxibustion and Traditional Chinese Medicine. Through these efforts, the hospital has expanded the awareness of the efficacy of Traditional Chinese Medicine all over the world. It has also cooperated with more than 10 medical organizations from the United States, Japan and other countries. Over 1000 of the hospitals doctors, nurses and medical technicians have been sent to present lectures and to provide medical treatment to over 20 countries, including the United States, Japan, Germany, Korea and Yugoslavia.

---

**"It works! The doctors and nurses are wonderful."**
**Red E.**

---

First Teaching Hospital of Tianjin University of Traditional Chinese Medicine continually analyzes the ways that the hospital encourages science and technology that results in scientific research reports. Results of these reports are now being used in the clinical treatments of patients throughout the world. The Dan Qi Pian Tan Capsule, developed by academician Shi Xuemin, is currently being marketed as a commercial medicine.

Now called NeuroAid™, this is a medicine which was historically developed in China as traditional Chinese medicine to help stoke patients achieve enhanced rehabilitation. Neuroaid is indeed a natural preparation made from carefully selected natural components which are abstracted in a proprietary standard process. Traditional Chinese medicines are typically made of cocktails of natural abstracts that physicians assemble for their patients. For each intake, the cocktail has to be boiled at home to obtain a decoction that the patient drinks. Beyond the obvious convenience issue of having to boil the ingredients three times a day – there is a more fundamental issues of consistency over time and geographies to ensure repeated efficacy and absence of side effects to guarantee the targeted therapeutic effects. Neuroaid has been fully standardized over the years by ensuring that the raw ingredients are consistently selected from the same sources, its manufacturing is handled with stringent quality process and controls

Neuroaid has undergone important clinical trials; these trials are being published in the west by the team at Moleac. They establish the absence of side effects as well as efficacy in providing patients with a strong impact on recovery. Patients taking Neuroaid have 2.1 more chances to achieve independence than patients not taking Neuroaid during the first six months which follow their stroke onset. It has shown important effect in these systematic trials on the motor functions.

With the lack of therapeutic options in the West to support recovery, Neuroaid has triggered huge interest from the clinicians in the west and there are actually several trials in western hospitals, evaluating the exact impact of Neuroaid on all the components of rehabilitation. CHIMES is a large trial now implemented by Neurologists in Asia is evaluating the additional benefits of Neuroaid if started within the first 48h after the stroke, over a duration of 3 months. With the result of CHIMES, Neuroaid may become a systematic post stroke treatment around the world to support faster and fuller recovery by 2010. By then Neuroaid cost will be picked up by many of the insurers.

Still until 2010, there will be another 1.5 million stroke in the USA, and it would be very frustrating not to be able to access Neuroaid, nor to be able to benefit from the full array of treatments available and proven to support recovery. I am happy that Moleac has not limited its work to clinical effort a per the usual pharmaceutical industry approach, but has strived to make Neuroaid available as soon as possible to sufferers around the world.

It first made Neuroaid available in the Republic of Singapore in 2006 and through their web site(www.neuroaid.com) started shipping to patients around the world. At the time of printing, this has enabled patients in over 25 countries to benefit from Neuroaid. Still even though the Chinese Pharmacopeia has been used for thousands of year, it lacks stystematic endorsement in many countries. In order to increase the reach of Neuroaid benefits to US patients with a local product, Moleac has come up with a dietary supplement formulation for the US market. Neuroaid10 (www.neuroaid10. com), is a simplified formulation of Neuroaid with all its major ingredients and benefits from the same high quality sources, processed in the same high quality manufacturing, available locally in the US.

Ruth has experienced personally the benefits of this medication and has been excited at its release and availability to the public at large. "I've seen hundreds of patients benefit from the use of Neuroaid and I'm thrilled it can now be obtained throughout the world."

Over 300 other traditional Chinese medicines such as Zhong Feng Bolus and Bao He Powder are known to have unique curative results and have has been documented and published. The Hospital affiliated Pharmaceutical Factory and the Health Material Factory, established according to modern GMP international standards, has created tremendous social and economic benefits. The factories have become the firm foundation of a modern Industrial group that combines Medicine, Education, Scientific Research and Industry in the production of traditional Chinese medicines.

# What exactly is Traditional Chinese Medicine (TCM)

## Types of Treatment

Traditional Chinese Medicine combines a number of therapies to provide the best environment for the body to heal itself. The easiest way to describe it is to visualize a doctor who puts a cast on a broken arm. He does not heal the arm, the body does. He simply provides the best environment for healing to occur.

## Acupuncture

The utilization of acupuncture needles in the hands, wrists, arms, head, neck, face torso, legs and feet. This treatment typically utilizes as few as 6 needles and as many as 60. The needles remain in for 20 minutes and the treatment is done twice daily.

## Chinese Massage

Done only by a doctor this is an aggressive and therapeutic massage. It may include legs, arms back and torso and usually lasts from 30-40 minutes.

## Chinese herbal medications

Several Chinese herbs and medications may be prescribed including a daily IV. Additionally, currently prescribed medication can be taken.

## Cupping

The application of glass cups to remove toxins and increase circulation in the body.

## Herb Soaks

These include herb soaks of the arm, leg or entire torso. The affected limb is placed into hot water and herbs are applied for at least 10 minutes.

## Steam Therapy

This includes the application of steamed herbs on the limbs or back for periods of time to include, but not exceed, 20 minutes.

## Heat Therapy – Moxibustion

This includes, but is not limited to, various heat therapies and the application of heat through the use of herb sticks and burning herbs on needles.

# What is Acupuncture?

## Definition

Acupuncture is one of the main forms of treatment in traditional Chinese medicine. It involves the use of ultra thin needles that are inserted in the body at very specific points. This process adjusts and alters the body's energy flow into healthier patterns, and is used to treat a wide variety of illnesses and health conditions.

## Purpose

Acupuncture has been recommended as an effective treatment for over forty medical problems, including stroke, arthritis, allergies, respiratory conditions, gastrointestinal disorders, gynecological problems, nervous conditions, and disorders of the eyes, nose and throat, and childhood illnesses, among others. Acupuncture has been used in the treatment of alcoholism and substance abuse. It is an effective and low-cost treatment for headaches and chronic pain, such as problems like back injuries and arthritis. It has also been used to supplement invasive Western treatments like chemotherapy and surgery. Acupuncture is generally most effective when used as prevention or before a health condition becomes acute, but it has been used to help patients suffering from cancer and AIDS. Acupuncture is limited in treating conditions or traumas that require surgery or emergency care (such as for broken bones).

## Origins

The original text of Chinese medicine is the Nei Ching, The Yellow Emperor's Classic of Internal Medicine, which is estimated to be at least 2,500 years old. Thousands of books since then have been written on the subject of Chinese healing and its basic philosophies spread long ago to other Asian civilizations. Nearly all of the forms of Oriental medicine which are used in the West today, including acupuncture, shiatsu, acupressure massage, and macrobiotics and have their roots in Chinese medicine. It is said that acupuncture developed when early Chinese physicians observed unpredicted effects of puncture wounds in Chinese warriors. The oldest known text on acupuncture, the Systematic Classic of Acupuncture, dates back to 282 A.D. Although acupuncture is its best known technique, Chinese medicine traditionally utilizes herbal remedies, dietary therapy, lifestyle changes and other means to treat patients.

In the early 1900s, only a few of the Western physicians who visited China were fascinated by acupuncture, but outside of Asian-American communities it remained virtually unknown. Then, during 1970s, Richard Nixon became the first U.S. president to visit China. On Nixon's trip, journalists were amazed to observe major operations being performed on patients without the use of anesthetics. Instead, wide-awake patients were being operated on with only acupuncture needles inserted into their bodies to control pain. During that time, a famous columnist for the New York Times, James Reston, had to undergo surgery and elected to use acupuncture instead of pain medication. He wrote convincing stories on its effectiveness.

## Why China for TCM?

In considering China for treatment, it is helpful to remember that this is a Chinese Hospital in China and not an American facility. Clients will encounter a different culture in China and unfamiliar protocols. To maximize benefits received, it is suggested that a client follow their Chinese doctor' advice and treatment regime. The client may not always understand why they do things differently, but results speak volumes.

It is helpful to keep in mind that TCM is slow medicine. It is not the same as taking a pill  and getting instantaneous results. TCM heals the brain first. The body  follows. It is important that a client remain positive and focused while allowing the body to relax and heal. One of the most common misconceptions is that more is better. Sometimes more is just more! Relaxation and rest are ways that the body heals  as many who have had treatment find. Te goal is to provide the best environment for maximum healing.

**Types of Treatments**

When a person becomes a patient of TCM they are involved in more than acupuncture. TCM treats the entire body. Chinese medicine views the body as a small part of the universe, and subject to universal laws and principles of harmony and balance. Chinese medicine does not draw a sharp line, as Western medicine does, between mind and body. The Chinese system believes that emotions and mental states are every bit as influential on disease as purely physical mechanisms, and considers factors like work, environment, lifestyle and relationships as fundamental to the overall picture of a patient's health. Chinese medicine also uses very different symbols and ideas to discuss the body and health. While Western medicine typically describes health in terms of measurable physical processes made up of chemical reactions, the Chinese use ideas like yin and yang, chi, the organ system, and the five elements to describe health and the body. To understand the ideas behind acupuncture, it is worthwhile to introduce some of these basic terms.

## YIN and YANG.

According to Chinese philosophy, the universe and the body can be described by two separate but complimentary principles, that of yin and yang. For example, in temperature, yin is cold and yang is hot. In gender, yin is female and yang is male. In activity, yin is passive and yang is active. In light, yin is dark and yang is bright; in direction yin is inward and downward and yang is outward and up, and so on. Nothing is ever completely yin or yang, but a combination of the two. These two principles are always interacting, opposing, and influencing each other. The goal of Chinese medicine is not to eliminate either yin or yang, but to allow the two to balance each other and exist harmoniously together. For instance, if a person suffers from symptoms of high blood pressure, the Chinese system would say that the heart organ might have too much yang, and would recommend methods either to reduce the yang or to increase the yin of the heart, depending on the other symptoms and organs in the body. Thus, acupuncture therapies seek to either increase or reduce yang, or increase or reduce yin in particular regions of the body.

## CHI

Another fundamental concept of Chinese medicine is that of chi (pronounced chee, also spelled qi). Chi is the fundamental life energy of the universe. It is invisible and is found in the environment in the air, water, food and sunlight. In the body, it is the invisible, vital force that creates and animates life. We are all born with inherited amounts of chi, and we also get acquired chi from the food we eat and the air we breathe. The level and quality of a person's chi also depends on the state of physical, mental and emotional balance. Chi travels through the body along channels called meridians.

## THE ORGAN SYSTEM

In the Chinese system, there are twelve main organs: the lung, large intestine, stomach, spleen, heart, small intestine, urinary bladder, kidney, liver, gallbladder, pericardium, and the "triple warmer," which represents the entire torso region. Each organ has chi energy associated with it, and each organ interacts with particular emotions. As there are twelve organs, there are twelve types of chi which can move through the body, and these move through twelve main channels or meridians. Chinese doctors connect symptoms to organs. That is, symptoms are caused by yin/yang imbalances in one or more organs, or by an unhealthy flow of chi to or from one organ to another. Each organ has a different profile of symptoms it can manifest.

## THE FIVE ELEMENTS

Another basis of Chinese theory is that the world and body are made up of five main elements: wood, fire, earth, metal, and water. These elements are all interconnected, and each element either generates or controls another element. For instance, water controls fire and earth generates metal. Each organ is associated with one of the five elements. The Chinese system uses elements and organs to describe and treat conditions. For instance, the kidney is associated with water and the heart is associated with fire, and the two organs are related as water and fire are related. If the kidney is weak, then there might be a corresponding fire problem in the heart, so treatment might be made by acupuncture or herbs to cool the heart system and/or increase energy in the kidney system.

The Chinese have developed an intricate system of how organs and elements are related to physical and mental symptoms, and the above example is a very simple one. Although this system sounds suspect to Western scientists, some interesting parallels have been observed. For instance, Western medicine has observed that with severe heart problems, kidney failure often follows, but it still does not know exactly why. In Chinese medicine, this connection between the two organs has long been established.

**Intensity and Focus**

When one enters the hospital it is as a patient . A patient is  focused on improving  health and overall disabilities. Acupuncture will be given by the leading TCM doctors in China. These doctors utilize a specific style of acupuncture that has been developed for stroke and is very effective.

**"I witnessed many who were receiving help and showing improvement. They all had their eye on that ball. I also received improvement. Thank you for all you do to help others."**

**Joe C.**

### Environment

When one enters the hospital as a patient, the environment and culture that a client enters into is Chinese. As such it is important to embrace the differences. An attitude of openness will aid in healing.

Ruth often tells people that she had an advantage as the first and only American There were no others to distract her, so she found that having clear focus and lack of distractions helped treatment and healing.

## The Aimin Weight Loss Hospital

The Aimin hospital is a leader in weight loss and hosts a very successful and proven fat reduction program. Developed by Mr. Lidong Shi in the 1990's, the 'Shi' fat reduction methodology has helped many people suffering from obesity as well as those who may just have a little weight to loose. Clients at the hospital were all treated on as inpatients to maximize weight loss.

Aimin's motto is:
"Serve society, develop and better ourselves and in doing so, help to create better health and well being for others."

The program itself is a combination of calorie controlled nutritional meals, acupuncture and regular exercise because at Aimin our aim is not only to assist our client in losing weight but to discipline and teach our clients the importance of healthy living by changes in their eating patterns, eating healthy food, and the involvement of regular exercise.

The Aimin Program is based on the principles of Traditional Chinese Medicine (TCM). TCM has three forms of treatment, Acupuncture, Herbal Medicine and a sophisticated system of Massage. It is worth noting that the World Health Organization (WHO) has acknowledged acupuncture as effective for the treatment of many conditions, obesity being one of them.

The treatment at Aimin is holistic including Acupuncture, Herbal Medicines, Massage, a Calorie controlled diet and regular exercise. At Aimin the treatment of acupuncture assists in the weight reduction process by

- Increasing the metabolic rate
- Assisting in the effective burning of excess fat
- Regulating the endocrine system
- Significantly improving or in many cases reversing obesity related illnesses
- Suppressing appetite

## Acupuncture

For this treatment fine stainless steel needles are placed into specific points on the torso, abdomen, thighs, legs and sometimes arms. Acupuncture mobilizes blood and moisture in the body to invigorate muscles, nerves, glands and organs. Some people find acupuncture completely painless. Others feel a slight pinch followed by numbness. It is not unknown to experience sensations of tickling, aching warmth or heaviness. Whatever the physical sensation, insertion of the needles is rarely painful and usually produces relaxation and a slight elevation of spirit. Needles stay inserted typically for 30 minutes. Once removed, needles are discarded immediately and new disposable needles are used for each new acupuncture treatment.

Aimin has a schedule of activities. These activities form the basis of our program and assist the client in forming new and healthy lifestyle patterns. In doing so, the client not only achieves the desired weight loss success but is also is on the way to understanding and maintaining their weight loss for the rest of their lives. This principle is the success of the Aimin program, fat reduction, desired weight loss and maintenance for life.

Some of the activities in the program include: walking, working out at a gymnasium, badminton, a variety of aerobic classes, basketball, swimming, excursions and other outdoor activities. Clients admitted to Aimin are expected to routinely do three exercise sessions per day. Our fitness experts and sports coaches supervise all sessions and monitor all clients. Clients are expected to perform only to their fitness level, and advance only when their fitness and health allows it.

Calorie controlled nutritious meals are prepared by the hospital chefs. These meals are prepared according to the Aimin fat reduction program for all inpatients and staff. The meals are served canteen style and not individually to inpatients or staff. The chefs and kitchen staff are happy to accommodate any client that has specific dietary requirements.

## Success stories:

Meng Qing Gang
Age: 21 years old
Country of Residence: China, Harbin
Date treatment began: 17 June 2000

I am 1.79m (5' 10") tall and weighed 265kgs (584 lbs) when I was first admitted to the Aimin Fat Reduction Hospital. Because of my weight I was often teased at school such that I stopped attending classes altogether.

On the first day of my treatment, after going through a medical examination, the hospital found out that apart from being severely obese, I was also suffering from heart disease, acanthosis nigricans (hyper pigmented, warty lesions of the axillae and perianal body folds), erysipelas (infectious skin disease characterized by redness, swelling etc and fatty liver.

Following 30 days of treatment, my weight reduced to 216.8kgs (477 lbs). On September 24, 2000, I was awarded in Shanghai the Guinness Record for having lost the most amount of weight in the shortest time span. To date, I had lost a total of 80kgs (176 lbs) in 100 days. On April 3, 2001 I weighed 128.9kgs (284 lbs). As a result of the dramatic weight loss, the medical conditions I had showed signs of improvement.

On the first anniversary since being admitted to hospital, I weighed 105kgs (231 lbs). By September 2001 I was officially discharged from the hospital having then weighed 90kgs (198 lbs). Since that time I have either fully recovered from all the medical conditions which I suffered from, or all signs and symptoms were now indicating normal levels.

To date my weight still maintains at the 90kgs (198 lb) level. During the treatment, I have learned the importance of watching how much and what I eat and doing daily exercise. I believe that this is the reason that I am able to maintain my weight.

---

J. Huang
Age: 14 years old
Country of Residence: Tianjin China
Date treatment began: July 2004
Weight before Treatment: 152.5kgs (335 lbs)
Height: 1.72m (5' 8")

My parents were extremely concerned about my severe obesity. Not only was I being teased at school, but also I had severe learning difficulties. I lacked concentration and I was always tired and lethargic. Walking around the playground was difficult and I was always out of breath even when walking short distances.

My parents had heard of many success stories and they knew that this was the right decision for me. I too, like other severely obese people, suffered from many ailments that were a result of my obesity, and I had double chins and no one could see my neck. Clothing me was very difficult, so my mother resorted to making clothes for me.

My waist measurement went from 152cm (60") to 85cm (33"), eight months after treatment I have reached a weight of 73kgs (160 lbs) which is the correct weight from my height. I lost an astounding 79.5kgs (175 lbs). I now eat normally, and my skin has contracted very well because of my age. I now wear standard clothing, and enjoy running, jumping and many other sporting activities. I now enjoy reading, studying and learning, and am looking forward to going back to school. I can now even see my neck.

I am very happy that my parents did the best for me, and I am grateful to them and to the Hospital. I have been taught to eat properly, when to eat, how much to eat, and the importance of dong exercises.

B. Zaidah Age: 29 years old
Country of Residence: Singapore
Occupation: Customer Service Consultant
Date treatment began: 3rd April 2003
Weight before Treatment: 150.5kgs (331 lbs)
Height: 1.73m (5' 8")

I had been struggling to deal with my weight problem for the past 10 years. I had tried going to the gym, taking medications, starving, but nothing worked for me at all.

I became interested in Aimin's weight loss program after reading about their most celebrated case – China's Meng Qing Gang who reduced his weight from 265kgs (584 lbs) to 90kgs (198 lbs).

During my stay in the hospital, the physicians tailored a comprehensive treatment program for me. It includes daily acupuncture sessions, physical exercises as well as a well-balanced diet plan.

When I was discharged from hospital on 21 September 2003, I had managed to shed 65.5 kgs. (144 lbs.). I felt good and a lot more energetic than before. My overall health condition also improved dramatically. The treatment has enlightened me on the importance of a healthy eating habit and lifestyle.

# 4

# 康复治疗
# RECUPERATION & REHABILITATION

Along with medically prescribed therapies, variety of activities will be made available during your recuperation. These activities are designed, not only to aid in the recovery process, but also provide a Chinese cultural experience.

## Paper Cutting

Begun between 206 BC and 221 AD, this is one of China's most popular folk arts. Paper cuttings are traditionally made on red paper. Red is used because the Chinese believe that red is a lucky color. The figures on the paper cuts are often dragons, birds, people, flowers, or Chinese characters. The paper cuts can be cut and glued onto a homemade card or gift to make it special.

## Tai Ji

180 million people worldwide practice Tai Ji every day. Tai Ji is an exercise that helps the body accumulates energy. Its emphasis is on deep breathing and uses mental imagery. Tai Ji integrates mind and body and relieves stress. Slow dance-like movements create balance, flexibility and calm and twenty minutes a day provides health benefits.

## Chinese Yoga Or Qigong

Qigong is a set of techniques used to increase vitality and longevity as well as help to achieve optimum health and inner peace. Qigong consists of a series of breath, gentle motions and relaxation.

# Journaling

Journaling is an easy and powerful way to accelerate personal development, to keep a detailed, personal musing during your medical tourism experience, and to gain insights you might not otherwise see.  It's a great method, too, for sharing your China medical experience with family and friends.

---

**"Great news I can get on the tip of my toes something I couldn't do before. GOD IS GOOD."**
**Olive G.**

---

# Chinese Language Skills

Take this opportunity to improve your ability to communicate in Chinese.  Learn to speak in basic phrases and feel more comfortable in one of the world's largest countries.

# Calligraphy

The word calligraphy means elegant handwriting.  It is the art of skilled penmanship and more.  Before the printing press was invented, this was the method used for printing books.  Learn this beautiful art and use it for brush writing and to make hand made invitations. Chinese calligraphy has a long history dating to 4000 years ago. No one can tell exactly when Chinese written language appeared.

# Chinese Needlework

An art over 3000 years old, Chinese needlework is used to accent accessories, on clothing and in framed art.  Learn the basic stitches of this form of embroidery art. Folk artists embroider flowers, birds, mountains, water, characters and animals with needles and lines. The work is lovely and vivid and abounds in decoration. Modern needlework can be classified into two types: appreciative needlework and applied needlework.

# 5

# 旅游在中国

# Traveling in China

Traveling in China is an exotic experience. Whether you are just flying to Beijing  or going on a mini holiday prior  or after your treatment, China is a country of variety, mystery and intrigue.

Most train stations and all airports have English-speaking personnel.  China Connection will meet the client upon arrival and arrange English-speaking tour guides for those who want or need them.

It is important to note that many locations only have European toilets available. For those of you who are new to this, they are at floor level and require squatting. Working with China Connection avoids this. Our staff can inform clients of the locations where handicapped accessible western style toilets can be found.

Money can also be a source of challenge. Many locations only take cash and while it is suggested that the client arrive with some local currency, all cities have a Bank of China ATM that accepts a VISA cash card and allows one to draw out Yuan (RMB) the local dollars. Exchange rates can be as good as 7.5 Yuan to 1 dollar or down to 7 Yuan to 1 dollar. The calculator that China Connection provides is invaluable. Use it to show values to pay for purchases even if one can't speak the language.  Chinese shopkeepers know this and on the street everything is negotiable. Start bargaining at 50% of the asking price.  Many times the Chinese escort can get a better deal if they know what the client wants.

You will find that traveling in China is a wonderful and enjoyable experience. The people are pleasant and helpful and any perceived language barrier can be overcome with a smile and hand gestures. Everyone you meet is willing to help and you will find a few well learned Chinese phrases (even if spoken badly) go a long way!

With this in mind we have listed a few of the many places there are to visit in China. You'll fall in love with the country, its people, places, culture and food. Many of these locations are explained in detail and others are listed to provide you basic information. Once you have been assigned a Chinese client manager they can provide you with an abundance of information about any of these locations.

We have contracted with one of the largest and best tour agencies in China to provide the best opportunities to our clients that wish to travel within China. Here are just a few reasons to book with our agency:

- Better Pricing in China
- Chinese know China
- Access to VIP Service
- Known Heath Travel Advantages
- English Travel Guide Access
- Personal Tours (not groups that are cancelled)

# Historical Relics

## The Great Wall

The Great Wall of China is one of the wonders of the world. Just like a gigantic dragon, the Great Wall winds up and down across deserts, grasslands, mountains and plateaus, stretching approximately 6,700 kilometers (4,163 miles) from east to west of China. With a history of more than 2000 years, some of the sections of the great wall are now in ruins or have entirely disappeared. However, it is still one of the most appealing attractions all around the world because of its architectural grandeur and historical significance.

The Great Wall was originally built in the Spring, Autumn, and Warring States Periods as a defensive fortification by the three states: Yan, Zhao and Qin. The Great Wall went through constant extensions and repairs in later dynasties. In fact, it began as independent walls for different states when it was first built, and did not become the "Great" wall until the Qin Dynasty. Emperor Qin Shihuang succeeded in his effort to have the walls joined together to fend off the invasions from the Huns in the north after the unification of China. Since then, the Great Wall has served as a monument of the Chinese nation throughout history. A visit to the Great Wall is like a tour through the history backwards.

The construction of the Great Wall drew heavily on the local resources for construction materials, was carried out in line with the local conditions under the management of contract and responsibility system. A great army of man power, composed of soldiers, prisoners, and local people, built it. The construction result demonstrates the manifestation of the wisdom and tenacity of the Chinese people.

---

**"Without Ruth we would not have gone and without her we would not have gotten the care that we received."**
**Dale L.**

---

The Great Wall as we see today was constructed mostly during the Ming Dynasty. It starts from Shanhaiguan Pass in the east to Jiayuguan Pass in the west traversing provinces of Liaoning, Hebei, Beijing, Tianjin, Shanxi, Inner Mongolia, Ningxia, Shaanxi and Gansu.

Following a forty-five day long survey of 101 sections of the Wall in different provinces, the China Great Wall Academy reported on December 12, 2002 that the forces of nature and destruction at the hand of mankind brought about the gradual reduction of its extent with the result that less than 30% remains in good condition. The Academy has called for greater protection of this important relic.

The Great Wall has long been incorporated into Chinese mythology and popular symbolism. The most beautiful of several legends is about the collapse of a section of the Great Wall caused by Meng Jiangnu, who cried bitterly over the death of her husband in the construction of the Great Wall.

This legend has been spread widely through textbooks, folk songs and traditional operas.

If you prefer to see the wall in a relatively natural state, visit Simatai, 110km northeast of Beijing. This part of the Wall is the best choice, for it is still in its original state without being developed into a popular tourist attraction due to its distance and little public transportation options.

## Qin Terra-cotta Army in Shaanxi (Xi An)

The Terra Cotta Warriors and Horses are the most significant archaeological excavations of the 20th century. Work is ongoing at this site, which is around 1.5 kilometers east of Emperor Qin Shi Huang's Mausoleum, Lintong County, Shaanxi Province. It is a sight not to be missed by any visitor to China.

Upon ascending the throne at the age of 13 (in 246 BC), Qin Shi Huang, later the first Emperor of all China, had begun to work for his mausoleum. It took 11 years to finish. It is speculated that many buried treasures and sacrificial objects had accompanied the emperor in his after life. Array in Pit1, Xian Terra Cotta Warriors Museum A group of peasants uncovered some pottery while digging for a well nearby the royal tomb in 1974. It caught the attention of archaeologists immediately. They came to Xian in droves to study and to extend the digs. They had established beyond doubt that these artifacts were associated with the Qin Dynasty (211-206 BC).

The State Council authorized to build a museum on site in 1975. When completed, people from far and near came to visit. Xian and the Museum of Qin Terra Cotta Warriors and Horses have become landmarks on all travelers' itinerary.

Pit3, Xian Terra Cotta Soldiers Museum Life size terracotta figures of warriors and horses arranged in battle formations are the star features at the museum. They are replicas of what the imperial guard should look like in those days of pomp and vigor.

The museum covers an area of 16,300 square meters, divided into three sections: No. 1 Pit, No. 2 Pit, and No. 3 Pit respectively. They were tagged in the order of their discoveries. No. 1 Pit is the largest, first opened to the public on China's National Day, 1979. There are columns of soldiers at the front followed by war chariots at the back.

Terra Cotta Warriors and Horses Museum, Xian, ChinaNo. 2 Pit, found in 1976, is 20 meters northeast of No. 1 Pit. It contained over a thousand warriors and 90 chariots of wood. It was unveiled to the public in 1994.Archaeologists came upon No. 3 Pit also in 1976, 25 meters northwest of No. 1 Pit. It was the command center of the armed forces. It went on display in 1989, with 68 warriors, a war chariot and four horses.

Over 7,000 pottery soldiers, horses, chariots, and even weapons have been unearthed from these pits. Most of them have been restored to their former grandeur.

The Terra Cotta Warriors and Horses is a sensational archaeological find of all times. It has put Xian on the map for tourists. It was listed as one of the world cultural heritages.

**Banpo Village Remains in Xi An**

Banpo Museum, Xian: The Banpo Museum is located in the eastern outskirt of Xian City, Shaanxi Province. As the first museum at the prehistoric site, it was built at the base of the excavations of the Banpo site. Since it opened to the public formally in 1958, two million people have visited it.

The Banpo Site is a typical Neolithic matriarchal community of the Yangshao Culture dating back about 6,000 years. At that time, the Banpo people used tools made primarily of wood and stone. Women, the crucial labor force, were responsible for making pottery, spinning, and raising the family, while men fished.

The first Exhibition Hall is about the unearthed relic exhibitions consisting of the First Hall and the Second Hall. The showpieces in this two halls are primarily production tools and domestic tools used by the primitive Banpo people, including axes, chisels, sickles, and stone and pottery knives from which we can have a general picture of the production activities of the Banpo people thousands of years ago. In addition, artwork and adornments here reflect the social life, culture, art and inventions of the period.

The Site Hall is about 3,000 square meters (about 0.7 acre) and contains residential, pottery making and burial section. And among the three, the residential section is the main part of the site, including the huts, kilns and tombs of the primitive residents. All these present us an outlook of the aboriginal village life

## Peking Man Site in Beijing

Zhoukoudian, about 50 kilometers (31 miles) southwest of Beijing, was a natural habitat of human ancestors about 700,000 years ago. To some extent, this is the cradle of Chinese civilization. In this charming and mystical land, Peking man left its footprints. Today, the remains and site provides a good opportunity for tourists to explore the primitive life of our human ancestors.

The Peking Man Site is situated in the Dragon Bone Hill near Zhoukoudian. Since 1921, eight sites of ancient human remains have been discovered. Twenty-six localities where high concentrations of fossils were found have been excavated. One hundred eighteen kinds of animal fossils and over 100,000 stone wares have been unearthed. These fossils and remains serve as evidence of the existence of humanoid species 500,000 years ago in Zhoukoudian.

Three representative remains exist: the Peking Man Site, the Upper Cave Man Site and the New Cave Man Site. In 1921, a cave was discovered at Zhoukoudian. Archaeologists confirmed it as the habitat of Peking Man. Today, it is called Locality One or Apeman Cave. In 1929, the discovery of a complete skullcap fossil by a Chinese Paleontologist, Pei Wenzhong, caused excitement around the world. The skullcap fossil could be traced back 500,000-700,000 years ago, proving the existence of Sinanthropus. This discovery serves as reliable and convincing evidence for the theory of evolution. Since then, Zhoukoudian has become known as the 'Home of Apeman'. Decades of scientific work and excavation revealed many skeletal fossils of the ancient Peking Man, stone and bone implements and ash residues.

The Upper Cave Man Site was discovered in 1930, and was excavated in 1933. It is located above the Apeman Cave near the peak of the Dragon Bone Hill. The cave is about 4 meters (13 feet) high and 5 meters (16 feet) wide. Three complete skullcap fossils and many other fossils were discovered here. Around the skeletons the powder of red hematite was also discovered. Other finds include bone needles, animal teeth and the remains of necklaces that were used as ornaments. These remains prove the utilization of animal furs to make clothes and to dress themselves and to keep warm. According to scientific research, the Upper Cave Man lived about 18,000 years ago with their physical character being quite similar to that of modern man.

In 1973, the New Cave Man Site was found in Locality Four, 100 meters (328 feet) south to the Apeman Cave. The New Cave Man lived 100,000 years ago. The discovery of this site bridges the gap between Peking Man and Upper Cave Man, and the succession of Peking Man's evolution. One tooth, fossils of amniotes and other animal fossils were unearthed here.

In September 2005, over 100 animal fossils were discovered in Gezitang hall. Gezitang hall is located at the entrance of Apeman Cave. Archaeologists have confirmed that the fossils discovered are the remains of several species of ancient deer that lived in the middle Pleistocene period. Three teeth fossils, several antler and upper jawbones of the ancient deer were found.

In 1953, the Peking Man Site Museum was founded and opened to the public, exhibiting over 3,000 cultural relics. The exhibits are mainly composed of fossils of the Peking Man and other animal bones, demonstrating the origin of creatures in prehistory and the transition from ape to human.

## Sanxingdui Remians in Sichuan

Sanxingdui Museum in Chengdu, China Sanxingdui Museum is located in Northeast of Sanxingdu archaeological site, west of the famous cultural city of Guanghan, on the bank of Jian River (commonly called Yazi River), 40 kilometers (about 24.9 miles) north of Chengdu City. Covering an exhibition area of 4,000 square meters (about 1544.4 square miles), and opened in October 1997 this is a museum with excellent modern facilities. The cultural relics in the museum were unearthed from the Sanxingdui site. In order to know about the museum we should know more about the Sanxingdui site.

Sanxingdui is a cultural relic of the ancient Shu (Sichuan). It is an important  discovery which changed the people's understanding of ancient history and culture. If one wants to visit a place to know more about Chinese Shu (Sichuan) culture, make it this one, for the civilization shown by the cultural relics can be called a true wonder.

Chengdu Sanxingdui Museum in Sichuan, ChinaSanxingdui refers to three earth mounds at the site. Hence the site found here is called Sanxingdui Relic. The Relic area stretches for about 12 square kilometers (about 4.6 square miles), which is the largest, oldest Shu cultural relic in Sichuan. It is said that the Heavenly Emperor cast down three handfuls of earth which fell near the Jian River and became three earth mounds on Chengdu Plain. The three earth piles, described as three golden stars in a line, hence became known as Sanxingdui (three-star piles). Now affirmed by modern archeology, the three earth mounds of the Sanxingdui Relic are in reality the southern wall of an ancient city that was built of earth. There are two breaches in the city wall, after the collapse and subsequent erosion it became the three mounds we see today.

The discovery of the Sanxingdui Relic was a lucky chance. In the spring of 1929, a peasant found a piece of bright-colored jade whilst he was digging ditch. That was the catalyst to the discovery of a mysterious ancient kingdom;. subsequently, more than 400 jade items were excavated. Later, from 1933, systematic excavations and archaeological work of Sanxingdui Relic continued for half a century. The evidence of the excavation shows the development from late Neolithic Age (7000 BC-5000 BC) through to the late Hang (16th - 11th century BC) and early Thou Period (11th century BC - 711 BC).Sichuan - Chengdu Sanxingdui Relic, with more than 3,000-year history might even be the capital of ancient Shu. In the following decades, several generations of archaeologists worked in succession on the Sanxingdui site and found two sacrificial pits in 1986. With more than 1000 cultural relics unearthed, including a 142-centimeter (about 55.9 inches) long and 500-gram (about 31 drams) golden staff, a golden veiled head portrait, a 260-centimeter (about 102.4 inches) tall and 180-kilogram (about 396.8 pounds) bronze figure, also a big bronze mask with more than 10 centimeters (about 3.9 inches) bulging pupils and two ears spaced at 168 centimeters (about 66.1 inches) and a big Yuzhang (a kind of jade adornment of the leader of a tribe, the symbol of power). Some cultural relics are apotheosized and mysterious, some are realistic, and some primitive simplicity and all of them aroused worldwide attention.

The discovery of Sanxingdui Relic, is the centuries-old center of the ancient Shu on Chengdu Plain. Traditionally, archeology considered Shu as a closed area and without communications to the Central Plain (the most developed region in ancient China), but the cultural relics unearthed here have affirmed ancient Shu is no less developed than the Central Plain and it is even the most representative cradle of Chinese civilization in the upper reaches of the Yangtze River. So Sanxingdui Relic is a significant means to comprehend the development of history and culture in Sichuan, and even the southwest area of China as a whole, yet Sanxingdui is still enigmatic. The ancient Shu characters are one of the two or three unbroken characters. Some cultural relics cannot be named as the archaeologists have never seen them before.

Sichuan - Sanxingdui Museum in ChengduIn order to well preserve and display the cultural relics, the Sanxingdui Museum laid the foundation in 1992 and opened in October, 1997. The museum is divided into four sections, and displays more than 1000 pieces of cultural relics from Sanxingdui Relic and the two sacrificial pits of Shang Period, including gold plate, bronze ware, jade articles, pottery and ivory. Each of the four sections has its own theme.

Section 1 Splendor of Ancient Shu Culture.
The section is divided into five units. The first unit outlines the history of the ancient Shu and introduces the background of the ancient Shu. The next four units reflect skill, imagination and technical achievements of the Shu people through their handicraft techniques.

Section 2 Mystery of the Primitive Faith

The exhibition in this section focuses on human and divinity. It adopted the imitative real scene to show the mental world of Shu people.

Section 3 Exquisite Cultural Artifacts

More than 10 groups of cultural relics exhibited here are treasures that symbolize the Shu people's ever lasting spirit.

Section 4 Sanxingdui: Excavation and Study

This section is a scientific display that introduced the impact of the Sanxingdui Relic overseas, the discovery and excavation of the site, the vital position of Sanxingdui Relic in academic study, that reflect all facets of Sanxingdui Relic.

For the large groups of tourists all year around, a new Exhibition Hall was opened on May Day in 2004, covering an exhibition area of 7,000 square meters. The exhibition in this hall is a complex display of jade articles, gold plate and pottery, with the old Exhibition Hall specializing in bronze wares.

**Ancient City of Loulan in Xinjiang**

One of the great mysteries in Chinese history is the disappearance of the ancient city of Loulan. The city was located about 300 km (186.4 miles) northeast of Ruoqiang County, Xinjiang Uygur Autonomous Region and adjacent to another early city, Dunhuang in Gansu Province. Like

Pompeii in ancient Rome which drowned in a sea of volcanic ash, and transformed the once beautiful city into a barren and perilous desert landscape. This inexplicable event has whetted the curiosity of archaeologists and other scientists over the years. Tourists, too, have been intrigued by this site and many venture there despite adverse weather and terrain

Loulan was established as a kingdom in 176 B.C. and flourished for over 800 years. The city was like an oasis traversed by a limpid river and situated next to a bountiful lake. The city had a population of over 14,000 including an estimated 3,000 soldiers guarding the safety of the kingdom. Many residents made a living fishing and hunting. As one of the major stops on the old Silk Road, the city was a center for the trading of silks, teas, fruit and jewels with the inland. Merchants also used Loulan as a stopover in their travels. The kingdom was booming economically while serving as a peaceful environment for its citizens and visitors.

Roughly around the year 630, Loulan suffered a natural disaster of epic proportions. Due to unceasing deforestation, raging sandstorms covered the region, rerouting the waterways transformed the city into a desert wasteland. To this day, the terrain is barely navigable as there are severe weather fluctuations. In the summer, the temperature has been known to shift from below 0 degrees C. to over 30 degrees C. from the night to the daytime. The region is extremely arid and continues to be subjected to frequent wind and sand storms.

Conditions are so harsh that the area has become known as the 'Death Sea.'

Only in recent years have archaeologists ventured into Loulan. Because of the dangerous environment, some actually have lost their lives. However, those that were able to conduct a successful dig found priceless treasures. The store of cultural relics included stone and jade tools and stone arrowheads dating back to the Neolithic Age (10,000 BC-5,000 BC). They also found manuscripts from the Han Dynasty (206 BC-220 AD) as well as silk, pottery, bronze ware, glassware, and ancient currency. So rich were these troves that researchers from around the world have dubbed this area 'Treasure Land of the Desert' and 'Museum Left by History.'

Perhaps the most famous discovery at the Loulan site is the Sanjian Fang, This a three-room building is said to be the yamen of the area's governor, and has a pagoda with 10.4 m. (34.12 feet) high, the tallest building in the city. Also discovered was a woman mummy, the called 'Loulan Beauty', in the Loulan ancient tomb ditch. The corpse is still intact after over three thousand years.

Travel Tips: Because of the difficult elements, Loulan is also known as 'the forbidden zone.' Bring lots of water, warm clothes, necessary medicines, handi-wipes and eye drops. Be prepared for high temperatures and dust. The road to the ancient city is extremely difficult and it is advised that visitors travel in groups. Visitors should also be reasonably fit. There are sightseeing buses in Ruoqiang County, but they cannot enter the archaeological site. If you want to go to the location of the cultural relics, you will need to either walk or ride a camel.

## Dawenkou Remains in Shandong

## Ruins of Guge Kingdom in Tibet

Located in the Ngari Region, Tibet Autonomous Region, the Ruins of Guge Kingdom are the Old Summer Palace of Tibet. While these ruins were once an imperial estate which fell into disrepair after the civil revolt and the invasion of the allied armies of eight foreign countries, the Guge kingdom also encountered civil strife and foreign attacks which fragmented the once prosperous state. However, the legendary kingdom hasn't been totally lost as much can be learned about it from its remains.

Established in about the 10th century, the Guge Kingdom was founded by one branch of descendants of a nearby crumbled Kingdom. It was ruled by about 16 kings with armies of tens of thousands of soldiers during the over 700 years in which it flourished. Then in the 1660s, conflicts resulting from power disputes within the imperial family emerged which engendered restlessness in society and induced civil uprisings. To win power in the disordered state, the brother of the king asked the ruler of the neighboring country Ladakh (the present Kashmir) to send his army to help. This army overthrew and conquered the kingdom. Only years later was power returned to Tu Lin. During its lifetime, the Guge Kingdom played an important part in the economic and cultural development of Tibet. The kingdom advocated Buddhism, and many versions of this religion were created here and their teachings were spread into the heart of Tibet. The kingdom also served as a major center for Tibet's foreign trade.

The Ruins of Guge Kingdom now extend around the sides of a mountain more than 300 m. (984 ft.) high. Explorers have found over 400 rooms and 800 caves here, as well as some fortresses, secret paths, pagodas, arm storerooms, granaries and all kinds of burial places. Except for some temples, all the roofs of the rooms have collapsed, leaving only the walls. The ruins are surrounded by a city wall and a fortress marks each of the corners. Palaces, temples and local residences are distributed from the top to the bottom and the only routes are secret roads to lead to the top, a layout designed to indicate the supremacy of the king and to ensure the safety of the palaces. Due to its great research value, the Ruins of Guge Kingdom have been listed under the first group of Cultural Relics of National Importance under the Protection of the State.

From this cave near Ruins of Guge Kingdom, over thirty mummies has been found. Perhaps the most interesting aspects of the Ruins are the five temples and palaces – the White Temple, Red Temple, Samsara Temple, Imperial Palace, and Assembly Palace. Many inscriptions, statues and murals are displayed inside these. The most complete and valuable artifacts remaining are the murals, which are  pictures of Sakyamuni, the king, queen, prince and other royal servants. Beside, in the sanctuary pictures of the cultivation of male and female Esoteric Buddhas can be found. The margins are painted with dozens of nude Dakinis. The colors and lines of the murals can be compared with those of the Mogao Caves in Dunhuang City, Gansu Province. Most of the statues here are golden and silver Buddhist statues, among these the Silver Eyes of Guge

## Silk Road

China's vast western region is accessible to travelers along the classic Silk Road, although historically, the trade route was never called such until a German geographer gave it that romantic name in the late 1800s. In AD 200, this transcontinental route linked the Roman Empire in the west with the imperial court of China. Trade along the route was carried on by foreign traders who belonged to neither of the two old empires.

Before the discovery of the sea route to India, the Silk Road was the most important connection between the East and West.  Its last great era was during the time of the Mongol Empire. This ancient trade route starts in the old capitals of Luoyang and Xian (then called Chang'an), reaches the Yellow River at Lanzhou, skirts westward along deserts and mountains before dividing into three routes at the oasis of Dunhuang.  Ancient travelers left behind many historical records and invaluable relics.

## Yin Ruins in Henan

In 1899, in Xiao Tun Village of Anyang City, Henan Province, villagers found many tortoise shells and bones carved with letters and symbols, which unveiled to the world Yin Xu, an ancient city with a long history and splendid culture. Since then this place has become of great interest to worldwide archeologists interest to archaeologists,. The inscriptions have proved to be the earliest written characters of human beings, the Oracles.

About 3,300 years ago, one emperor of the Shang Dynasty (16th - 11th century BC) moved his capital city to Yin, which is today's Anyang city, and since then Yin has been the capital city for more than 250 years. Today Yin Xu has proved to be the earliest remains of an ancient capital city in written record.

Covering a grand area of 24 square kilometers (more than 9 square miles), Yin Xu had a palaces district, civil residences district, tombs district and workshops district, divided into two parts by the Heng River in the city.

The large-scale excavation in Yin Xu continuous the last century. Besides the 150, 000 pieces of oracles, abundant bronze ware has been excavated, and among them, Simuwu Ding, a 4-legged bronze cooking vessel is the biggest and heaviest bronze ware ever found worldwide. Apart from oracles and bronze ware, people have also excavated much pottery ware and jade.

## Forbidden City in Beijing

Lying at the center of Beijing, the Forbidden City, called Gu Gong in Chinese, was the imperial palace during the Ming and Qing dynasties. Now known as the Palace Museum, it is to the north of Tiananmen Square. Rectangular in shape, it is the world's largest palace complex and covers 74 hectares. Surrounded by a six meter deep moat and a ten meter high wall are 9,999 buildings. The wall has a gate on each side. Opposite the Tiananmen Gate, to the north is the Gate of Devine Might (Shenwumen), which faces Jingshan Park. The distance between these two gates is 960 meters, while the distance between the gates in the east and west walls is 750 meters. There are unique and delicately structured towers on each of the four corners of the curtain wall. These gates afford views over both the palace and the city outside. The Forbidden City is divided into two parts. The southern section, or the Outer Court, was the place the emperor exercised his supreme power over the nation. The northern section, or the Inner Court was where he lived with his royal family. Until 1924

---

**"I'd given up hope of ever having a productive life again before I went to China. Today, I not only can work full time, but am pain free for the first time in years. China Connection and TCM is truly a gift."**

**John L**

---

when the last emperor of China was driven from the Inner Court, fourteen emperors of the Ming dynasty and ten emperors of the Qing dynasty had reigned here. Having been the imperial palace for some five centuries, it houses numerous rare treasures and curiosities. Listed by UNESCO as a World Cultural Heritage Site in 1987, the Palace Museum is now one of the most popular tourist attractions world-wide.

Beijing - Forbidden City Construction of the palace complex began in 1407, the 5th year of the Yongle reign of the third emperor of the Ming dynasty. It was completed fourteen years later in 1420. It was said that a million workers including one hundred thousand artisans were driven into the long-term, hard labor. Stone needed was quarried from Fangshan, a suburb of Beijing. It was said a well was dug every fifty meters along the road in order to pour water onto the road in winter to slide huge stones on ice into the city. Huge amounts of timber and other materials were freighted from faraway provinces. Ancient Chinese people displayed their considerable skills in building the Forbidden City. The grand red city wall  has an 8.6 meters wide base reducing to 6.66 meters wide at the top. The angular shape of the wall is impossible to climb. The bricks were made from white lime and glutinous rice while the cement is made from glutinous rice and egg whites. These materials make the wall extraordinarily strong.

Forbidden City in Beijing Since yellow is the symbol of the royal family, it is the dominant color in the Forbidden City. Roofs are built with yellow glazed tiles; decorations in the palace are painted yellow; even the bricks on the ground are made yellow by a special process. However, there is one exception. Wenyuange, the royal library, has a black roof.  It was believed black represented water  and could extinguish fire.

Nowadays, the Forbidden City, or the Palace Museum is open to tourists from home and abroad.

## Yuanmingyuan in Beijing

The Old Summer Palace which is also known as the Ruins of the Yuanmingyuan (the Garden of Perfection and Light) is located northwest of Beijing and to the east of the Summer Palace. The Garden was first constructed in the year of 1709 during the reign of the Emperor Kangxi of the Qing Dynasty (1644-1911). Over the next 150 years of the Qing Dynasty, this Garden was expanded to be a large-scale Chinese emperors' private pleasure garden, covering a total area of 350 hectares (over 864 acres).

The  Old Summer Palace consists of three parts - Yuanmingyuan, Wanchunyuan (the Garden of Blossoming Spring) and Changchunyuan (the Garden of Eternal Spring). These three gardens are often referred to as one common name: Yuanmingyuan. Hundreds of scenic spots in the Garden are made up of exquisitely constructed halls, pavilions, chambers, kiosks, earth and rock hills, rivers and ponds, and exotic flowers and grasses from different parts of the country. Indeed, it embodies the essence of Chinese ancient landscape gardening.

Old Summer Palace (Yuanmingyuan), Beijing, China To be distinct from other traditional Chinese Gardens, the garden construction and horticulture of Yuanmingyuan is a harmonious blend of typical Chinese scenery and western architecture. The more famous scenic spots include, for example, the Grand Waterworks, the Throne for viewing the Waterworks and the Labyrinth. No wonder Yuanmingyuan was also called the 'garden of gardens' or the 'Versailles of the East' in Europe during that era. Yuanmingyuan was also an imperial museum that collected a large number of books, treasures and cultural artifacts. However, a large number of these collections were plundered by the Anglo-French Allied Forces in 1860, at the same time as the Garden was burnt down. Now, most of these historical curiosities are displayed in the other countries museums, including the British Museum; Bibliotheque Nationale de France; Metropolitan Museum of Art, New York City, USA Oslo Museum of Applied Art and so on.

The vast majority of the remaining scenic spots were destroyed in the 1980's, but under the due protection of the ruins of Yuanmingyuan a park has been established on the ruin site. Visitors can imagine the former grandeur of the Old Summer Palace from the crumbling walls and ruins. What's more, there is also an opportunity for visitors to view the complete picture of Yuanmingyuan in its 'heyday' in the exhibition hall. The reconstruction of some of the original structures and scenic spots provides people with a lovely place to relax.

## Mountain Resort of Chengde in Hebei

The Mountain Resort of Chengde, located at Chengde City Hebei Province, is the largest imperial garden in modern China. It covers a total area of 564 square kilometers, and is twice as large as the Summer Palace in Beijing. In the Qing Dynasty, it took 89 years (1703 ~ 1792) to complete. The emperors Kangxi and then Qianlong were in charge of this project.

The Mountain Resort, also a summer resort, is an important location of wonderful scenery and pleasant climate. Grand palaces, delicate temples, peculiar mountains, abound. Tourists will have the choices of walking, hiking, climbing, riding and boating inside the garden.

The Palace Area and Scenic Area are the main parts of the Mountain Resort.

Palace Area: Palaces in China conjure up pictures of majesty and splendor The architectural style of the palace is unique, and similar to the resident houses in North China. Black bricks and gray tiles, rock steps and the courtyard covered with old pine trees look peaceful and elegant.

The palace area is made up of the Main Palace, Pine-Crane Hall, Pine Soughing Valley and East Palace. In the past, the Qing emperors lived there and dealt with some government affairs. It was the second center of the imperial palace at that time. The Forbidden City in Beijing was the first one. Emperors held celebrations in the mountain resort.

Scenic Area -- Lake Zone, Plain Zone and Mountain Zone

Lake Zone: Water gives everything infinite vitality and energy, so the scenery of the lake zone sparkles like a diamond in the Mountain Resort. Lying in the southeast of the resort, the lake zone has nine lakes and ten islands, such as Half-moon Lake, Mirror Lake, Silver Lake, Inner Lake and others, around which are the main scenic areas. Weeping willows along the banks and green waves rippling on the water make a wonderful picture.

Plain Zone: Going north, tourists arrive at the plain zone. Facing the palace wall on the east with the mountains rising to the west, this area are covered with grassland and woods. The plain zone is divided into three parts: an arboretum to the east with 28 various Mongolia tents; to the west is a piece of grassland where one can ride horses, and temples and other buildings lie to the north. Scenery on the plain zone is simple and serene.

Mountain Zone: There are four great valleys from north to south: Pine-cloud Valley, Pear Valley, Pine Valley and Filbert Valley. Enjoy the mountains, undulating hills, flourishing woods, steep peaks, gurgling streams and white waterfalls.

Each year in the summer, the Qing emperors would come and live there for about five to six months. They could not only discuss the court affairs with the ministers, but also vacation. Nowadays, once summer starts, many people think of the Mountain Resort of Chengde and travel there to spend their vacations.

## Ancient City of Jiaohe in Xinjiang

One of the world's architectural wonders hides in Yarnaz Valley, 10 kilometers (6.2 miles) west of Turpan. Like a willow leaf, the ancient city of Jiaohe (Yarkhoto) with a history of 2300 years lies between two rivers on a loess plateau atop a cliff of over 30 meters (98.4feet). The largest, oldest and best-preserved earthen city in the world, Jiaohe, is 1,650 meters (5,413 feet) by 300 meters (984 feet) at its widest; with an area of 220,000 square meters (2,368,168 square feet).

Jiaohe was the capital of the former Cheshi State. An Indian proverb says, "intelligence is bound to exist where two rivers meet". Jiaohe, meaning , where two rivers meet, is such a place. According to historical records it was home to 700 households, 6500 residents plus 865 soldiers.

The Ancient City of Jiaohe in Turpan, Xinjiang Jiaohe distinguishes itself from other ancient cities owing to three features. First, it had only two city gates, the South and East Gates. The main South Gate vanished long ago, leaving a huge breach. The East Gate cut by the cliff was virtually non-existent. Second, the city faces cliffs on three sides, so there are no city walls as commonly seen in other ancient cities. Third, all the buildings were dug from dirt, and wood was rarely used.

The central avenue, 350-meters (1148.3-feet) long, runs north from South Gate, separating the city into three parts; namely, residences for common people, temples, and residences for aristocrats.

To the west of the avenue, low buildings with sparse small temples were residences for commoners, while the higher ones in the east were for aristocrats and troops. At the end of the avenue stands a large well-preserved Buddhist temple, Jiaohe Temple, with an area of 5,000 square meters (53,824 square feet).

Xinjiang - The Ancient City of Jiaohe in Turpan The relics we see today featured Tang Dynasty ( 618-907) architectural style. Houses were dug downward from the earth, and as no house gates faced the streets, military defense was apparently a priority.

At the end of the 8 Century, the city was tossed into the reigns of the Turpan, Hui, and Mongols. Residents fled from the destroyed city continuously until in the beginning of the fourteenth Century and the city was abandoned, as was its glory and prosperity of over 2000 years. Miraculously, owing to the arid climate and remote location, the ancient city of Jiaohe remains intact, leaving us a rare example of an earthen castle.

# Mountains

### Five Most Famous Mountains :

Mt. Taishan in Shandong
Mt. Hengshan in Hunan
Mt. Hengshan in Shanxi
Mt. Huashan in Shaanxi
Mt. Songshan in Henan

### Four Buddhist Holy Mountains :

Mt. Jiuhuashan in Anhui
Mt. Putuoshan in Zhejiang
Mt. Emeishan in Sichuan
Mt. Wutaishan in Shanxi

### Famous Taoist Holy Mountains:

Mt. Wudangshan in Hubei
Mt. Qingchengshan in Sichuan
Mt. Longhushan in Jiangxi
Mt.Qiyunshan in Anhui

### Other Famous Mountains in China :

Mt. Huangshan in Anhui
Mt. Yandangshan in Zhejiang
Mt. Laoshan in Shandong
Mt. Tianshan in Xinjiang
Mt. Qingxiu in Guangxi
Mt. Tiantaishan in Zhejiang
Mt. Lushan in Jiangxi

Mt. Wuyishan in Fujian

Mt. Maijishan in Gansu

Mt. Jingganshan in Jiangxi

Mt. Fanjingshan in Guizhou

Jade Dragon Snow Mountain in Yunnan

## Waters

### Rivers:

Yangtze River

Li River in Guangxi

Nanxijiang River in Zhejiang

Qin Huai River in Jiangsu

Yellow River

Grand Canal

Fuchunjiang River in Zhejiang

### Lakes:

Dongting Lake in Hunan

Taihu Lake in Jiangsu

Shouxi Lake in Jiangsu

East Lake in Hubei

Jingpo Lake in Heilongjiang

Poyang Lake in Jiangxi

West Lake in Zhejiang

Qinghai Lake in Qinghai

Qiandaohu Lake in Zhejiang

## Beaches:

### Beidaihe Beach in Hebei

Beidaihe Scenic Spot, the famous summer resort, is located in the southwest of Qinhuangdao City. Its coastlines, seaside attractions and convenient transportation all make it a popular destination for travelers. Beidaihe Scenic Spot is situated in the warm temperate zone, with a damp monsoon climate and four distinct seasons, is neither too hot in summer nor too cold in winter. Therefore, it is suitable for all year round travel, though, the best time to visit is from May to October.

The long coastline to its south has soft sand and sea water of moderate salinity, making it an excellent place to sunbathe and swim. Many modern holiday villages and public bathing places have been established where one can taste local snacks and delicious seafood, ride in a speedboat, or relax by ballroom dancing.

In the central area of the scenic spot is a great attraction called Tiger Rock Park. It has many huge rocks looking like a herd of tigers. Standing on any of the rocks is a great spot for photography.

To the east another famous attraction is the Yingjiao Stone - a twenty-meter (66 feet) steep rock like an eagle perched on the cliff. Because groups of doves nest in the cracks there, it is also called Dove Nest Park. The Yingjiao Pavilion on the top is known as a place to watch the sunrise.

The pine-covered Lianfeng Hill, which backs on to Beidaihe beach, comprises two peaks, the east peak and the west peak. Taking the secluded path you can reach Wanghai Ting (Seaside Pavilion) at the top of the hill, to appreciate the vast sea and the scenery around the mountain. At the foot of Lianfeng Hill is a beautiful park named Lianhuashi (Lotus Stone Park) because of the many unexpectedly huge lotus shaped stones.

## Beihai Silver Beach in Guangxi

Beihai Silver Beach lies in the south of Beihai City, 10 kilometers (about 6 miles) away from city center. The beach stretches 24 kilometers (about 15 miles) from west to east with a width between 3 and 3,000 meters (3-3,281 yards). It is reputed to be the best beach in China for its advantages of even length, fine, white sand, clean, warm water and gentle waves. The natural advantages of the beach gives it the reputation of the "Eastern Hawaii" and is regarded as a resort for beach bathing and sports in the southern region of China. It is a preferred choice for sanatoriums in view of its clean and fresh air.

There are three sections of the resort, Beihai Silver Beach Park, Beihai Beach Park and Hengli Ocean Sports and Entertainment Center, as well as the villas and off shore and restaurants.

In the Beihai Silver Beach Park, one can find houses related to musical instruments, chess, books and pictures in the east part. In the middle section are sea ports and beach zones while in the west is a marine biology museum, a children's swimming pool and an open air dance floor. There are flourishing flowers and trees growing on the square and over 30 pavilions of various styles around the square. In addition, tourists can appreciate the songs of rare foreign birds, folk customs, Russian customs, and take part in parachute jumps over the water.

## Dadonghai Beach in Hainan

One of the most popular tropical seaside holiday areas in Hainan Province is located 3 kilometers (about 1.9 miles) southeast of downtown Sanya, between Mt. Tuziwei and Mt. Luhuitou. Dadonghai has a crescent-shaped beach 2.3 kilometers long (about 1.4 miles) and clear blue sea, sunshine, white sand and green trees creating a beautiful location in the Torrid Zone.

The famous beach is ideal for diving, beach sports, bathing and sunbathing. And as it has all amenities to support a seaside tourist location, including a large shopping square on the shore, amusement companies and a famous dive company that can provide scuba diving, ship diving, seabed strolling, speed boat, motorboat, luxury yacht, sail boat, ocean fishing, beach sports and underwater photography. This location is renowned for water activities in Sanya and throughout China.

Dadonghai and has spring-like weather all year round. The water temperature is about 20C degrees even in winter.

## Qingdao Beach in Shandong

Qingdao Seashore Scenic Area, located in South of Qingdao, integrates mountains, sea waters and architecture. This scenic area is along the coastline, extending 25 kilometers (16 miles) from east to west, with an area of 8.4 sq kilometers (3.2 sq miles) on land and 5 sq kilometers (2 sq miles) in the water. In 1982, it was listed among the finest national scenic spots.

Qingdao Seashore Scenic area is an open scenic spot, consisting of six sections: Qingdao Bay, Huiquan Bay, Taiping Hill, Badaguan Scenic Area, the Eastern New City Area and Shilaoren Tourist Holiday Resort. The major scenic spots include Zhan Bridge, Luxun Park, Small Qingdao Island, Xiaoyu Hill, Baihua Garden, Huiquan Square, May 4th Square (Wusi Square), Music Square, Yan'erdao Park, No.1, No.2, No.3, No.6 Bathing Beach, Binhai Sidewalk. These picturesque spots display the charm and scenery of the Qingdao seashore.

The six major scenic areas with distinctive characteristics mirror the unique seashore scenery. Qingdao Bay, located in the southwest of Qingdao, is a concentration of scenic spots and the most important part of Qingdao Seashore Scenic Area. Huiquan Bay Scenic Area distinguishes itself from others in Qingdao by its picturesque scenery. Every summer, tourists flock to the Huiquan Bay to enjoy sunbathing and the surrounding scenery of its beautiful bathing beaches. Taiping Hill Scenic Spot is characterized with its abundant plants and animals. With many well-equipped villas, Badaguan Scenic Area has become an ideal place for vacationing and sightseeing renowned for the distinctive architectural complex. The New City Area, built in 1990s, fully illustrates the results of the modernization of Qingdao. It has become the city's center of finance, commerce, culture and entertainment.

Shilaoren Tourists Holiday Resort is rich in both natural and cultural resources. This scenic area is enclosed by three hills in the north, west and east. In the south lies a broad and smooth beach covered with fine sand. Hills, sea, flowers, reefs with the cultural sceneries such as the Dolphin Performance Museum and Beer Town make this area charming both naturally and culturally.

The blue sea, gentle breezes, azure sky, green trees, red roofs and yellow walls make Qingdao outstanding and unique. Among its many sightseeing opportunities, May 4th Square is a landmark building. It covers an area of 100, 000 sq meters (119,599 sq yards), surrounded by towering trees and green lawns dotted with blooming flowers. The theme sculpture on the square, "The Wind of May" is like a burning torch, symbolizing vigorous development in Qingdao.

Walking along the Binhai Sidewalk and Seashore Sightseeing Road to enjoy the distinctive seashore scenery, tourists may imagine themselves walking in a fairy-tale land. Every year, tens of thousands of tourists from home and abroad are drawn to Qingdao Seashore Scenic Area.

## Yalong Bay in Hainan

Yalong Bay boasts unparalleled beauty. The 7.5-kilometer (4.7-mile) long, crescent-shaped bay with an area of 18.6 square kilometers (about 7.2 square miles) is one of the famous scenic spots in Hainan Province.

With the average temperature a pleasant 25.5C all year-round, Yalong Bay is situated in the southernmost part of Hainan Province, 25 kilometers (about 15.5 miles) away from the tropical seaside tourist city, Sanya. The area boasts endless rolling hills, serene gulfs, clear blue sea and silvery sand beaches and is three times as long as any in Hawaii. Home to several well-preserved coral reefs with tropical fish of varied kinds, the ocean here is crystal clear, allowing visitors to view underwater sights up to 10 meters (33 feet) deep.

Yalong Bay boasts the five essential elements of modern tourism: sea, sands, sunshine, lush green plants and fresh air. In 1992, the Secretary-General of the World Tourism Organization once marked that this bay embraces the unique and unparalleled natural settings, sands, crystal sea water, endless seashore, unspoiled hills and pristine vegetation, making it a paradise for holiday travelers.

Surfing in the sea, Yalong Bay, Sanya. Because of the unbeatable environment, Yalong Bay Resort was authorized by the State Council in 1992. The unique state-level tourist resort is characterized by its tropical ambiance - the resort holds seaside parks, deluxe villas, conference centers, top-end hotels, golf-courses It is the first choice for people who conduct conferences.

In the center of Yalong Bay square stands a Totem Pole of 27 meters (about 88.6 feet), on which the God of Sun, and Gods of Wind, Rain, and Thunder as well as those legendary animals such as Dragon, Phoenix, Kylin and Fish are engraved. The design of this square embodies the Chinese civilization of 5,000 years and has received recognition in winning the Luban Prize, a prize awarded to the top level design of architecture in China.

With an area of 3,000 square meters (about 3,558 square yards), Shell Hall of Yalong Bay is located in the central square of the resort. And with the shell as its theme, the Shell Hall is a comprehensive exhibition hall combining exhibition and shopping.

In the north of Yalong Bay is the site of Butterfly Valley, which is classified into five halls that present species of butterflies in China and other countries as well.

## Springs:

Baotu Spring in Jinan
Hupao Spring in Zhejiang
Baisha Spring in Hunan
Huishan Spring in Jiangsu
Huaqing Hot Springs in Shaanxi
Loubao Spring in Guizhou

## Waterfalls:

Huangguoshu Waterfall in Guizhou
Dalongqiu Waterfall in Zhejiang
Hukou Waterfall in Shaanxi
Nuorilang Waterfall in Sichuan

## Temples and Monasteries

White Horse Temple in Henan
Jinci Temple in Shanxi
Huayan Monastery in Shanxi
Famen Temple in Shaanxi
Dongguan Mosque in Qinghai
Labrang Monastery in Gansu
Songzanlin Monastery in Yunnan
Confucius Temple in Shandong
Id Kah Mosque in Xinjiang
Fuxi Temple in Gansu
Xiangguo Temple in Henan
Potala Palace in Tibet
Drepung Monastery in Tibet
Sakya Monastery in Tibet

Shaolin Temple in Henan
Baoguo Temple in Zhejiang
Yonghe Lamasery in Beijing
Hanshan Temple in Jiangsu
Po Lin Monastery in Hong Kong
Guiyuan Temple in Hubei
Lingyin Temple in Zhejiang
Hanging Monastery in Shanxi
Bright Filial Piety Temple in Guangdong
Qingyang Palace in Sichuan
Ta'er Monastery in Qinghai
Jokhang Temple in Tibet
Tashilhunpo Monastery in Tibet

## Natural Scenes

Jiuzhaigou Scenic Area in Sichuan
Yellow River Scenic Area in Henan
Zhangjiajie Scenic Area in Hunan
Beidaihe Scenic Area in Hebei
Mt. Jiuhua Scenic Spot in Anhui
Mt. Wuyishan Scenic Area in Fujian
Mt. Emeishan Scenic Area in Sichuan
Huanglong Scenic Area in Sichuan
Wulingyuan Scenic Area in Hunan
Stone Forest in Yunnan
Mt. Lushan Scenic Area in Jiangxi
Mt. Huangshan Scenic Area in Anhui
Mt. Taishan Scenic Area in Shandong
Huangguoshu Scenic Area in Guizhou

## Mausoleums

Mausoleum of Yandi Emperor in Hunan
Mausoleum of Yu the Great in Zhejiang
Maoling Mausoleum in Shaanxi
Zhaoling Mausoleum in Shaanxi
Ming Tombs in Beijing
Ming Xiaoling Mausoleum in Jiangsu
Tomb of Wang Jian in Sichuan
Fuling Tombs in Liaoning
Zhaojun Tomb in Inner Mongolia
Hairui Tomb in Hainan
Tomb of Huo Qubing in Shaanxi
Tombs of Prince Jingjiang in Guangxi
Mausoleum of Huangdi in Shaanxi
Mausoleum of Emperor Qin Shi Huang in Shaanxi
Tomb of Crown Yide in Shaanxi
Qianling Tomb in Shaanxi
Tomb of Princess Yongtai in Shaanxi
Tomb of Crown Prince Zhanghuai in Shaanxi
East and West Mausoleums of Qing Dynasty in Beijing
Mausoleum of Genghis Khan in Inner Mongolia
Mausoleum of Dr. Sun Yat-Sen in Jiangsu
Mausoleum of General Yue Fei in Zhejiang

## Gardens

Summer Palace in Beijing
Mountain Resort of Chengde in Hebei
Grand View Garden in Beijing

Garden of the Master of the Nets in Jiangsu

Li Garden in Jiangsu

Classical Gardens of Suzhou

Canglang Pavilion in Jiangsu

Lion Grove in Jiangsu

Garden for Lingering in Jiangsu

Humble Administrator's Garden in Jiangsu

## Towers and Pagodas

Yellow Crane Tower in Hubei

Tengwang Pavilion in Jiangxi

Daguan Pavilion in Yunnan

Wangjiang Tower in Sichuan

Mapang Drum Tower in Guangxi

Big Goose Pagoda(Dayanta) in Shaanxi

Haibao Pagoda in Ningxia

Six Harmonies Pagoda in Zhejiang

Iron Pagoda in Henan

Yan'an Pagoda in Shaanxi

Yueyang Tower in Hunan

Zhenhai Tower in Guangdong

Jiaxiu Tower in Guizhou

Wenchang Tower in Guangxi

Dongpo Pavilion in Guangxi

Small Wild Goose Pagoda in Shaanxi

Wooden Pagoda in Ying County in Shanxi

Three Pagodas of Saintly Worship in Yunnan

Wanbu Huayanjin Pagoda in Inner Mongolia

Longhua Pagoda in Shanghai

## Ethnic Group Flavors

Mapang Drum Tower in Guangxi

Baimian Yao Village in Guangxi

Longsheng Yinshui Dong Village in Guangxi

China Folk Culture Villages in Guangdong

The Ethnic Relics Center in Guangxi

Chengyang Winds & Rain Bridge in Guangxi

National Ethnic Group Park in Yunnan

## Museums

Chongqing Museum

Hebei Provincial Museum

Hubei Provincial Museum

Jilin Provincial Museum

National Museum of Chinese History in Beijing

Shaanxi Provincial History Museum

Shanghai Museum

Luoyang Ancient Tombs Museum in Henan

Zhaoling Tomb Museum in Shaanxi

Banpo Village Remains Museum in Shaanxi

Ming Tombs Museum in Beijing

Sanxingdui Remains Museum in Sichuan

Beijing Art Museum

Museum of Qin Terra-cotta Warriors and Horses in Shaanxi

Western Han Nanyue King Tomb Museum in Guangdong

China National Silk Museum in Zhejiang

Museum of Ceramic History in Jiangxi

Macau Grand Prix Museum
Macau Wine Museum
Gansu Provincial Museum
Hotan District Museum
Hunan Provincial Museum
Nanjing Museum
Palace Museum in Beijing
Shandong Provincial Museum
Xinjiang Regional Museum
Luoyang Stone Carving Museum in Henan
Qianling Tomb Museum in Shaanxi
Xianyang Terra-cotta Museum in Shaanxi
Forest of Stone Steles Museum in Shaanxi
Dalian Natural Museum in Liaoning
Beijing Natural History Museum
China National Tea Museum in Zhejiang
Aquatic Products Exhibition Center in Guangxi
Macau Maritime Museum
Hong Kong Space Museum

## Ancient Cities and Towns

Tongli Town in Jiangsu
Luzhi Town in Jiangsu
Wuzhen Town in Zhejiang
Nanxun Town in Zhejiang
Pingyao Old City in Shanxi
Xidi Village in Anhui
Zhouzhuang in Jiangsu
Mudu Town in Jiangsu

Xitang Town in Zhejiang
Jingdezhen in Jiangxi
Lijiang Old Town in Yunnan
Dali Old Town in Yunnan

## Grottoes and Caves

Mogao Caves in Gansu
Yungang Grottoes in Shanxi
Dazu Grottoes in Chongqing
Binglingsi Thousand Buddha Caves in Gansu
Leshan Giant Buddha in Sichuan
Longmen Grottoes in Henan
Maiji Caves
Three Immortals Buddhist Caves in Xinjiang
Kizil Thousand Buddha Caves in Xinjiang

## Local Resident Houses

Qiao's Compound in Shanxi
Siheyuan Courtyard in Beijing
Wang's Compound in Shanxi
Cao's Compound in Shanxi
Yongding Hakka Earth Building in Fujian
Ancient Residential House in Shexian County in Anhui
Chang's Compound in Shanxi
Cave-house in Northern Shaanxi
Qu's Compound in Shanxi
Naxi Residential House in Yunnan

# 6

# 归国
# 期待什么
# Going Home
# What to Expect

Whether going home or spending some time touring China it is important to be well enough along in recovery to travel. All too often, agencies and countries other than China discharge patients soon after surgery and have them check into a hotel with a private nurse. This is an uncomfortable choice at best. The China client will be asked to remain in the hospital until he is well enough to travel safely.

---

**"My son went to China for treatment as a completely disabled, pain- riddled 26 year old. China Connection offers not only offers hope and help, but healing. My son now lives a pain free, high energy life. I've gotten my son back. What other gift is better?"**

**Karen L.**

---

Most individuals choose to rest and use some of their recuperation time to learn new skills. We will work with clients to help them feel as ready to travel or tour, whatever their choice may be in addition, recuperation activates enrich the China experience.

Upon your arrival at home, plan on allowing a few days to rest and readjust to time changes.

Surgery and/or treatment will require slowly easing back into daily routine. As a client of China Connection a copy of *The 90 day Journey* workbook will be provided to assist in adjustment.

During the next thirty days, it may be tempting to try and see friends and extended family. The suggested formula is: one month of recuperation for each day in the hospital. It is important to continue the process of rest and recuperation, even though one has returned home and feels well.

# 7

# 如何把握现在
## HOW TO PROCEED

## Okay... what do I do now?

If you or someone you love is seeking treatment or surgery abroad then you owe it to yourself to pursue China as a destination. Whether you are facing Bypass surgery, knee replacement, an in-depth cardiac health check-up, rehab for stroke or treatment for migraines, with  technology, level of care, new facilities, talent and methods of treatment, there is no better place in the world to receive treatment and healing.

---

**"Wayne is a fine example of the success you offer and we are very thankful for all you have done to help both of us."**

**Carol G.**

---

Start by contacting the China Connection main office at 641-485-9667 or visiting them on- line at chinaconnection. cc (please note the .cc). You can receive information and an informational DVD for free by simply requesting it.

Then it's simply a matter of choosing your surgery or type of treatment, being assigned and working with a U.S. client manager, and deciding what you want to do during your recuperation or travel. China Connection will make the rest easy!

# 8

# 专业性
## TERMINOLOGY

# TERMINOLOGY OR GLOSSARY OF TERMS

ACAPUNCURE.  Application of slender, ultra thin needles for the purpose of healing.

ANGIOGRAM.  An x-ray technique used to measure blood flow and blood pressure in the coronary arteries.

ANGIOPLASTY.  Procedure performed to open narrowing in the coronary arteries.

ASSISTED HATCHING.  Procedure in which an artificial weakness is created in the shell surrounding the embryo.

BARIATRIC SURGERY.  General term for weight-loss procedures.

BREAST AUGMENTATION.  Surgical procedure to enhance the size of the breasts by using inflatable implants, usually filled with silicone or saline.

BREAST LIFT.  Surgical procedure to reshape sagging breasts.

CANDIDATE.  One chosen for something specified.

CARDIAC CATHATERIZATION.  A fine tube or catheter, is threaded from the groin to the heart.

CUPPING. Application of glass cups to remove toxins and increase circulation.

CT SCAN. A radiologic technique that selects a place in the body and blurs out structures above and below that place, leaving a clear image of the selected anatomy.

EKG. Electrocardiogram. A test that makes a graphic record of the electrical activity of the heart.

EYELID SURGERY. Surgical procedure to correct drooping upper eyelids and puffy bags below the eyes.

GALL BLADDER REMOVAL. The gall bladder, which stores bile, sometimes becomes obstructed or damaged and needs to be removed.

HERBAL INFUSION. Several herbs and medication and may be delivered through an IV line.

HERBAL SOAKS. Hot water and herbs mixed together and used, often on the arm, leg or torso. Soaks take at least ten minutes.

LIPOSUCTION. Procedure used to improve shape by removing exercise-resistant fat deposits with a tube and vacuum device.

HORMONAL THERAPY. Using the result of hormone blood tests, doctors prescribe a treatment regime to ensure that the woman has correct hormones to induce fertilization or to prepare the lining of the uterus to receive an embryo.

INTRACYTOPLASMIC SPERM INJECTION. A form of in vitro fertilization outside the body by injecting the sperm directly with a syringe.

INVITRO FERTILIZATION. Eggs are fertilized outside the body, then embryos are introduced into the uterus.
MEDICAL RETREAT. A period of withdrawal and privacy for the purpose a medical procedure.

MOXIBUSTION. Application of heat therapy through the use of heated, wrapped herbs rolled onto sticks or adding heated herbs to acupuncture needles.

MRI. A diagnostic tool that produces clear images of the body without the use of x-rays. MRI used a large magnet, radio waves and a computer.

PET SCAN. A noninvasive diagnostic tool that takes images of the human body by detecting tiny particles from radioactive material. May be used in conjunction with the CT scan.

PROTOCOL. Detailed plan of a medical procedure.

SIMS CARD. A portable memory chip use din some models of cellular phones.

STENT. A coiled wire, sometimes medicated, may be inserted into a narrowed coronary artery after angioplasty. The stent is used to keep the vessels open.

TCM. Traditional Chinese Medicine. Is a range if traditional medical practices developed in China over thousands of years.

TRANSUREATHRAL RESECTION OF THE PROSTATE. When this gland below the bladder becomes enlarged, often in older men, a partial or total resection (TURP) allows the bladder to function fully.

TUINA. A form of vigorous Chinese massage.

JOINT REPLACEMENT SURGERY. Surgically removing all parts of a damaged joint and replacing it with a new joint, called a prosthesis.

# 9

# 中文单词及短语

## HELPFUL CHINESE WORDS & PHRASES

## Chinese Words and Phrases
### Numbers

| | | |
|---|---|---|
| y ī | one | 一 / 壹 |
| è r | two | 二 / 贰 |
| s ā n | three | 三 / 叁 |
| s ì | four | 四 / 肆 |
| w ǔ | five | 五 / 伍 |
| liu | six | 六 / 陆 |
| q ī | seven | 七 / 柒 |
| b ā | eight | 八 / 捌 |
| ji ǔ | nine | 九 / 玖 |
| sh í | 10 | 十 / 拾 |
| b ǎ i | 100 | 一百 |
| qi ā n | 1,000 | 一千 |
| w à n | 10,000 | 一万 |
| l í ng | 0 | 零 |

### Dates

| | | |
|---|---|---|
| w ǔ | noon | 中午 |
| r ì | day | 天 / 日 |
| x ī ngq ī | weekday | 工作日 |
| yu è | month | 月 |
| ni á n | year | 年 |

### Directions

| | | |
|---|---|---|
| b ě i | north | 北 / 北方 |
| d ō ng | east | 东 / 东方 |
| n á n | south | 南 / 南方 |
| x ī | west | 西 / 西方 |
| zh ō ng | center | 中 / 中心 |

Verbs
sh ì    is                     是
y ǒ u   has                    有
z ǒ u   walk                   走

Pronouns
w ǒ    I                       我
n ǐ    you                     你
t ā    she/ he                 她／他
m é n  [plural]                复数

Nouns
sh ū   book                    书
r é n  person                  人
j ī ng capital                 首都
gu ó   country                 国家
y ǒ u  friend                  朋友

Others
y ī ng hero                    英雄
m ě i  beautiful               美丽
g è    [measure things]
b ě n  [measure books]
sh à ng up                     上
xi à   down                    下
w à ng towards                 向

How are You? -Ni Hao Ma        你好吗?

Also commonly shorten to Ni Hao.
通常也可以简称 "你好" 。

Thank You -Xie Xie. 谢谢

Very Good -Hen Hao. 很好

Ni Hao Ma? (How are you?) 你好吗?

Hen Hao (Very Good) 很好

No Good -Bu Hao. 不好

Ni Hao Ma? (How are you?) 你好吗?

Bu Hao (No Good) 不好

Very Expensive -Hen Gui 很贵

Don't want or No -Bu Yao 不要

This is beautiful -Hen Piao Liang 很漂亮

Taxi -De Shi 的士 / 出租车

Good Bye or See You Again -Zai Jian 再见

Excuse Me -Jie Guo 借过 / 请问 / 对不起 / 麻烦

Receipt -Fa Piao 发票 / 收据

I don't want -Wo Bu Yao 我不要

# 10

# 中国式礼仪

## CHINESE PROTOCOLS

# Protocols

Although China is essentially a group-oriented culture, it has a powerful tradition of individual responsibility and self-reliance. It is important to show proper respect for individuals. Hierarchy is demonstrated through humility and saving face. This kind of respect is shown by minimizing oneself. This, in the eyes of a Chinese citizen, raises one's esteem. It will be helpful for clients to know this when meeting doctors.

Clients may hear the word guanxi spoken and used in describing the quality of relationship between the China Connection staff at staff at your hospital. This refers to the relationship between individuals. Until one is brought into esteem in Chinese culture, relationships are formal and distant. When one earns respect and trust, good guanxi, occurs. China Connection has learned how important this is and has established good guanxi for clients.

Chinese are punctual and clients should be mindful of schedules, but will discover that once into a meeting or appointment, western styles of task-oriented behavior disappear and things will take the time needed to complete a task in spite of the clock. China's workday begins around 7AM and ends around 4PM.

Many of the Chinese staff at the hospital where one will be a patient speak English and are eager to improve their English. Although one is  be provided with a translator, it is recommended that clients take the time to learn some Chinese phrases in Chapter 7. It is a sign of respect to be able to speak a few words in the  native language

China is a non-touching culture. People often bow and exchange business cards rather than exchange handshakes, although they have become accustomed to this American way of greeting. It is acceptable upon meeting a Chinese person to begin by make eye contact,  then drop one's eyes and look toward the ground.

Anything that reflects a client's interests and hobbies are acceptable subjects of conversation. The Chinese love to talk about food! It is not wise to speak of politics, current events, or any controversial subject. Winking and whistling are considered vulgar. If a  doctor is formal in a meeting about health, consider this a sign of respect and reflection of the culture rather than personal distancing.  Once a staff member gets to know the client, formality is often relaxed.

---

**"I am truly thankful for our time in China!"**

**Kyle R.**

---

Never tip anyone. It is not done. Ever.  Tipping in China is offensive.

Street clothing should be selected so that one does not stand out.  Neutral colors work best. Any clothing that attracts attention is not acceptable.

Personal hygiene is very, very important. Wearing perfume is not popular and makeup and hairstyles should not be excessive. Moderation in wardrobe choice is good to remember when packing for your journey.

# 11

# 推荐参考
## REFERENCES

## BOOKS:

*Chinese Medicine, The Web That Has No Weaver*
by Ted J. Kaptchuk, Rider Publishing, 2001

*Out of The DARKNESS into The Light*
by Ruth E. Lycke, AuthorHouse, 2005.

*The 90 Day Journey*
by Ruth E. Lycke, AuthorHouse, 2008

*Things Chinese*
by DuFeibao, China Travel and Tourism Press, 2001.

## LINKS:

chinaconnection.cc
hopehelpandhealing.net
www.NeuroAid10.com

Printed in the United States
121218LV00001B/302/A

9 781434 354020